Exercise in a Bottle

As we like to remind people, "If exercise were a pill, everybody would take it." Expert panels from the American Heart Association, the American College of Sports Medicine, the Centers for Disease Control, and the National Institutes of Health all advise 30 minutes or more of moderate to intense physical activity on most days of the week. Yet, despite those recommendations and exercise's many benefits, only one in five adults gets the necessary amount of regular physical activity. Approximately 250,000 U.S. deaths per year (12 percent of all deaths) are due to health problems caused by lack of exercise. It can be difficult to begin an exercise program and sometimes even harder to stick with it. Take the following typical example.

Imagine that you just had a heart attack. As with half of those with coronary heart disease, the chest pains of your heart attack were your first symptom of heart disease. Leaving the hospital, you are anxious and worried that the problem will return. Maybe next time will be the "big one." In the hospital, you learned that regular exercise reduces the chances of another heart attack (see Chapter 9). Your doctors and the hospital staff encouraged you to join a supervised cardiac rehabilitation exercise program, which is paid for by your insurance. In this program, you and others with similar heart problems are watched closely during your workouts three to five times a week.

You would think that a recent brush with mortality and exercising in a safe, supportive atmosphere would provide plenty of motivation. Not so. At best, the chances are only 50/50 that you will be exercising after six months. So, why don't we all exercise, and what would help us be more physically active?

Under the best of circumstances, half of the people starting an exercise program drop out by six months.

I See Exercise in Your Future

One way that scientists have tried to help us get active is by comparing people who do and do not get regular exercise. Researchers figured that if they knew the differences between exercisers and nonexercisers, then they could concentrate on those differences to get us more active.

Findings were gathered from all types—young and old, men and women, Republicans and Democrats. Scientists found that if you are physically active, you are more likely to have certain characteristics. The more of these traits you have, the greater the likelihood you will exercise regularly. You can see how things add up for you by totaling your answers to the items in Table 2.1. Your score can range from a high of +17 to a low of –7. If you are not already exercising, the higher your total, the more likely you are to begin and stick with exercise in the future.

Unfortunately, the score is not a perfect indicator. We are too unique to have our behavior foretold so accurately. However, this quiz gives you a sense of how easy or difficult it may be for you to get on track with regular exercise. The higher your score, the greater your *readiness to change,* and the more likely you are to be successful with regular exercise. If your answer is less than 7, then you should ask yourself, "Why isn't my number higher?" and "What would it take to move the number up?" The single best question that indicates whether you will be able to successfully start exercising is shown in Table 2.2. Your answer measures your *self-efficacy,* or your belief in your ability to

---

TABLE 2.1   **Your Exercise Score**

Answer each question and add the points for your total score.

	Yes
I have exercised regularly in the past	+2
My spouse (or significant other) supports my exercising	+2
I participated in school athletics	+1
I have enough time to exercise	+2
My work is considered a blue-collar job	–2
I have a place to exercise	+2
I am a smoker	–2
I think I am overweight	–2
My friends support my exercising	+1
I have risks for heart disease (diabetes, high blood pressure, or high cholesterol)	+2
I feel healthy	+2
I am college educated	+1
I am more than 50 years old	–1
I enjoy exercise activities	+2
Your total score	_____

TABLE 2.2   How Would You Rate Your Exercise Self-efficacy?

On a scale of 1 to 10, how likely are you to stick with a program of regular exercise? (Circle your response)

1	2	3	4	5	6	7	8	9	10
Not going to do it				Chances are about 50/50					Sure thing that can't miss

---

exercise regularly. If you have a strong belief that you can do it, you usually can.

Most of us start an exercise program several times before we succeed. Still, it can be disappointing (and expensive) to join a health club and never go, or buy the latest exercise equipment only to have it collect dust. If your score is low, then your time might be better spent solving your road blocks, rather than deciding where to exercise. It is best to start your journey toward fitness with a full tank of motivation, so read on.

Do the words *regular exercise* sound like a lot of physical activity? Remember, any amount of exercise is better than nothing, and many of its benefits come with only 30 minutes of activity three times a week.

William was a 72-year-old man who was new to the clinic. He and his wife moved to the area following his retirement as head accountant for a northern California software firm. Although he felt well, he wanted to establish a place for his medical care. William's physical examination and laboratory studies confirmed his good health.

A decade ago, as his weight and blood pressure crept up, his doctor told him to "watch it" and advised exercise. He bought a book on running that came with a log for recording your mileage. Just as the text instructed, he began with short jogs and increased his distances slowly. When we saw him, he ran three to four miles each day. Since starting he rarely missed a day, rain or shine. His wife gave up asking him not to go running when the roads are icy.

While William might seem a little rigid and lacking in spontaneity, he enjoys his structured routine and takes pleasure in its consistency. It is hard to argue with success. He is the exception that proves the rule. He is just about the only person we know who "just did it." Most of us have to work at being physically active—experimenting with when to exercise, what to do, and how to fit it into our daily routine.

Making Changes

Changing a behavior is not a single event. It is a process with many steps along the way. Scientists have learned that a behavior has six stages. Figure 2.1 lists these as they relate to exercise, but the same six occur when you stop smoking, start eating a healthy diet, or change any other behavior. The stages are set in a loop, rather than a line, because forming (or breaking) a habit is usually not a one-way trip. As the saying goes, habits (both good and bad) are made to be broken, then remade, then rebroken, then remade—somewhat like New Year's resolutions. Most of us keep circling through these phases. Importantly, each stage of the journey requires something different. Knowing where you are allows you to focus your energy on what is needed to move you to the next stage. Like finding your way on a map, you need to know where you are to see how to get to the next destination. Table 2.3 lists the six stages and what actions are needed to move to the next step.

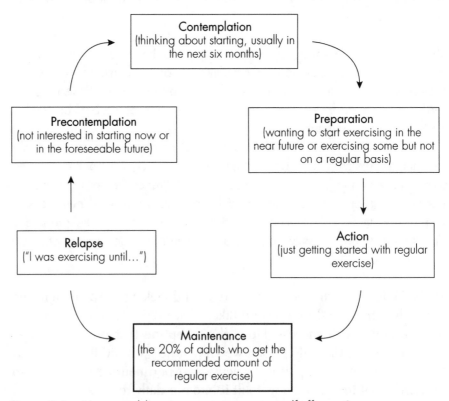

Figure 2.1   How would you rate your exercise self-efficacy?

TABLE 2.3 **Road Maps for Your Stage of the Journey**

In This Stage	You Probably Are Feeling	To Move to the Next Stage, You Need to
Precontemplation	There is no way that I am going to start exercising now or in the next six months. Check back with me later.	Learn more about exercise and its benefits. Correct any misperceptions about physical activity. For example, you might have the mistaken notion that you must exercise vigorously for its benefits, or that after age 60 it is too late to start exercising. Find out how regular exercise would benefit you. Which of the positive effects of exercise would you like to have? Feeling better, losing weight, strengthening your back, lowering your blood pressure? Explore available resources. If you decided to exercise, what facilities would be available? Is there a local gym, work-site fitness facility, or neighborhood track? What sorts of activity do you think you would like to do?
Contemplation	I'm thinking about exercising. I know it would be good for me, but I am not sure I can do it now. There is a lot on my plate already.	Congratulate yourself for taking the first steps. You are thinking about exercise. You should give yourself credit for any movement toward your destination, not just when you reach Maintenance. At this stage, you need to increase your commitment and confidence that you will succeed. It is not time to get specific about exercise and worry about which type of shoes to buy. You still are at the pep rally before the big game. You need to get pumped up. Can someone or something inspire you to exercise? Is there someone who could be your partner? Fill in the balance sheet in Table 2.4 to get more specific about your reasons for and against exercise. Ask yourself, "Which reasons are most important to me?" How have you changed other behaviors? Everyone has made changes—getting a job, marriage, parenthood, putting down the toilet seat. You have done more difficult things than finding a way to exercise. You can do this, if you put your mind to it.
Preparation	I want to be more physically active, and I am ready to get started.	Now is the time for specific advice about exercise. What are your options? What problems do you anticipate and how can they be solved? Who and what might help you?

TABLE 2.3 **Road Maps for Your Stage of the Journey** (continued)

In This Stage	You Probably Are Feeling	To Move to the Next Stage, You Need to
		Set goals you can achieve in the first two weeks of exercise. "Getting in shape" is too vague, and no one trains for a marathon in two weeks. Maybe your first goals are getting proper shoes and a calendar to record your progress. Each short-term goal you achieve keeps you on the right track.
		Writing down your exercise goals and your game plan for achieving them as an "exercise contract" can be helpful and reinforce your commitment (Table 2.5). After you have signed your name, the exercise agreement is binding in courts of tennis, squash, and basketball.
		If you plan to begin vigorous exercise, then you might need a stress test before you start your program. If you are older than 40 (for men) or 50 (for women), and/or have a major risk(s) for heart disease (high cholesterol, diabetes, high blood pressure, cigarette smoking, or strong family history of heart disease), check with your health care provider before beginning vigorous exercise. You need a preexercise evaluation. Chapter 9 discusses medical evaluations before exercising.
Action	I've been exercising regularly for a few weeks. I'm still working through road blocks and figuring out what works for me.	Reward yourself for your accomplishments. We are not that different from when we were six years old and motivated by gold stars. Rewards are not just for show. They help strengthen your program.
		Set new short-term goals and keep them realistic and achievable.
		Stimulus control means placing cues in your path that remind you about exercise. This could be the sneaker-shaped refrigerator magnet that encourages you to work out or the gym bag on your car's back seat that prompts you to exercise on the way home.
Maintenance	I've been exercising for more than six months, and it's become a habit. I miss it when I don't exercise, but it is still	Reward yourself for your accomplishments. Only one in five people is doing what you have done.
		Think about mixing in new types of exercise. Cross training and combining different physical activities

	You Probably	
In This Stage	**Are Feeling**	**To Move to the Next Stage, You Need to**
	difficult not to let other things get in the way.	helps avoid injuries and adds variety to your workouts.
		Anticipate what might make it harder for you to exercise. Avoid those situations when you can, and if you cannot avoid them, plan ways to work around them. Table 2.6 helps you think about barriers to exercise, and their solutions.
Relapse	I was doing well, until . . . . I'm trying not to be discouraged and plan to jump back into Action soon.	Almost everyone falls off the exercise wagon. It happens. Get over it and back at it. Maybe breaking your routine was unavoidable. What have you learned for next time?
		The task is to start around the "circle" again, rather than becoming discouraged and fixed in this stage. You did it before, and you can do it again.

**TABLE 2.3 Road Maps for Your Stage of the Journey** (*continued*)

The trip starts with the *precontemplation* stage. A precontemplator is someone who does not exercise and is not interested in starting. While we can imagine a person addicted to nicotine not wanting to stop smoking, it is hard to believe that someone does not want to exercise. Yet, 10 percent of inactive people feel that way. That probably does not include you, because you are reading this chapter. We are betting that most of you have moved past that stage and are at least in the Contemplation stage.

About 25 percent of nonexercisers are contemplators. If that is you, then you would like to be more physically active, but your exercise self-efficacy score (Table 2.2) is probably a 5 or less. When asked about regular exercise, your answer is, "I know I should exercise, *but.* . . ." For you, now might not be the best time to start an exercise program. Your chance of success is greater if you first move to the next stage by pumping up your resolve to be a regular exerciser. Table 2.3 lists ways for contemplators to move to the next stage.

If your exercise self-efficacy score is 6 or 7, then it is likely you are in the *preparation* stage. Join the crowd. A third of inactive people are here with you. You may have joined a gym, bought fitness equipment,

---

TABLE 2.4 **To Be or Not to Be an Exerciser (Your Health Is the Question)**

Complete the balance sheet for yourself. Which reasons are most important to you?

My Reasons for Not Getting Regular Exercise	My Reasons for Getting Regular Exercise
Samples: Don't like to sweat.	*Samples*: I'll be less anxious.
I'm a natural born klutz and seem to lack the gene for exercise.	My blood pressure could go down.
I can't find the time to exercise.	I'll be less of a "girlie-man."
I'm afraid of getting an injury.	My doctor might stop bugging me about it.

When it comes to regular physical activity, approximately 10 percent of people are in the Precontemplation stage, 25 percent are in the Contemplation stage, 30 percent are in the Preparation stage, 20 percent are in the Maintenance stage, and 15 percent no longer exercise regularly—the Relapse stage.

or found an exercise partner. Although you are not working out regularly, you are headed in the right direction.

If you have been exercising regularly for less than six months, then you are in the *action* stage. You have almost arrived and can claim your choice of names as a new action figure—Princess of Power, Road Warrior, Wild Man Sweating (you decide). The first six months are a critical part of your journey. It is during this time that you are most likely to fall into the *relapse* stage. Once you get past the six month milestone, you are in the *maintenance* stage.

Although the stages may look like numbers on a clock, that does not mean you will move through them at a steady speed. On this clock, time can stand still (or even reverse direction) in any stage. Of course, now you know what to do each step of the way. So, you should be traveling at double time toward your destination.

TABLE 2.5 **Contract Negotiations**

Whereas I, _____, being of sound mind, will begin a program to become of sound body by starting to exercise on _____ (date). I will exercise by _____ (name the physical activity), a minimum of _____ days per week, for at least _____ minutes each session, for the next _____ weeks. I will exhibit due diligence in the conduct of said exercise.

Exerciser: . . . . (the dotted line)

Witness: _____

Agreement made and entered this _____ day of _____, 20 ____ .

Ruth is 52 years old, and before two years ago, she never exercised regularly. When growing up, there were not many sports for young women. (Remember that women were not allowed to run a marathon in the Olympics until 1984.) Although physical education class was required in high school, Ruth remembered only once when she was made to sweat. On that warm spring day, the eleventh-grade girls ran one mile on the track. It seemed to take forever to finish. A friend fainted, and another classmate threw up. The experience was not repeated.

On her fiftieth birthday, Ruth resolved to start exercising. She had been bothered by an assortment of minor health problems, felt stressed, and could see herself sliding rapidly from middle to old age. She knew she needed to make some changes. She joined a gym and started riding the exercycle and attending step-aerobics. She saw the weight room but felt it was male territory. She was self-conscious and unfamiliar with the wide assortment of what appeared to be medieval torture devices (wasn't that why the men were groaning?). She was definitely out of her comfort zone.

Ruth is a school administrator, and her education background helped convince her to hire a personal trainer. Although initially thinking it self-indulgent, she liked being her trainer's main focus. She knew that professional athletes have a coach and a trainer. Shouldn't we nonathletes just starting to exercise get the same help? She also found that an appointment to exercise, when her trainer was expecting her, helped her be consistent. Her trainer showed her proper technique with the weight machines, and they designed a program to strengthen her back and upper body.

Today, Ruth is comfortable in the weight room. Before lifting weights, she shoots free throws. The repetitive motion helps her leave behind some of the tension from work and warms her up for exercise. Then she pumps iron. She likens the people in the weight room to children on a playground. Everyone is doing his or her own thing but enjoys the occasional interaction and the company of others on the playground.

There is no perfect exercise program. What seems to work for you today may not be right for others, and it might not be right for you a month from now. Today, exercise trainers are more available, and it is not just movie stars and rock musicians who can afford them. It is money well spent if it helps you develop and maintain your exercise program. Look for a trainer with an undergraduate degree in sport physiology, recreation, or health education, who is certified by a national organization. Avoid those selling nutritional supplements on commission.

Maintaining Your Change

Maintenance is the word used when you have changed a behavior. You have made it through the critical first six months when we are most vulnerable to losing the exercise habit. The trouble with the term is its suggestion that maintenance does not require any work on your part. Maintenance is not trouble-free driving between oil changes. Even after months of regular physical activity, your exercise program will need tune-ups.

Sometimes, it becomes more difficult to exercise. After many months, your fitness level will hit a plateau, and you will lose the positive reinforcement of seeing yourself improve. Remember, staying fit, even if you are not improving, makes you healthier. Over time, you may become bored with your exercise routine, or perhaps the weather changes, and you do not want to walk outside in the subzero temperatures. It may be time for swimming, enrolling in a tap-dancing class, or trying home workout videos.

Nearly all of us have breaks in our physical activity routines. That is, we relapse into our sedentary ways. Beating yourself up about it is not a beneficial training activity. What happened? Can you avoid this next time or alter your activities so you will not need to stop exercising? Table 2.6 lists some of the road blocks that you might experience and

TABLE 2.6 **Running through Road Blocks to Regular Exercise**	
Potential Road Blocks	**Ways to Go Around**
Samples:	*Samples:*
Weather turns too cold	Move it inside—home equipment, join a gym, mall walking?
Bored with the same old exercise route	Try a walkman and renting books on tape
Exercise partner moves away	Maybe a new training partner (either two- or four-legged)

examples of how others have broken through those barriers. Fill in Table 2.6 with your own road blocks and their potential solutions.

Avoiding Injury

Injuries can sideline anyone who exercises. You can reduce your chance of an injury by following the advice in Table 2.7. <u>Rule 1</u> is to not get too much of a good thing. Our muscles, tendons, ligaments, and bones are more likely to be damaged when we overexercise. For example, when your weekly running distance is greater than about 20 miles, the chance of injury climbs. To stay healthy, alternate among different types of exercise.

Cross training has nothing to do with working out while angry. It refers to combining different physical activities. Rather than walking or running each workout, mix in some days of cycling, weight lifting, and

---

TABLE 2.7   **Advice for Avoiding Injury**

1. Alternate among workout activities to avoid an overuse injury.
2. Allow your body time to adapt by not increasing your activity by more than 10% a week.
3. Pay attention to your body. If it hurts, don't do it. You may turn a minor problem into a bigger injury.
4. Use well-functioning equipment, good shoes, and appropriate safety measures to stay injury free.

---

racquet or team sports. Although the exercises differ, you still accumulate health benefits. By varying the stress on different parts of your body, you lower your risk of an overuse injury.

Rule 2 is to resist the urge to say that if a little is good, a lot is better. Often, we become impatient with getting into shape. Your body can make changes only so fast, and you will not speed it along by working out harder or longer. The rule of thumb is to increase your activity level by no more than 10 percent a week. So, if you are walking 10 miles one week, you would increase to only 11 miles (a 10 percent increase) the following week. This gives your body a chance to adapt to the new activity level, with less chance of an injury.

Rule 3 is to listen to your body when you exercise. You might think that athletes can block out what they feel while exercising. It is really the opposite; they usually pay more attention and are more alert for physical problems. For us, that translates to, "If it hurts when you do it, don't do it." The training credo should be, "No pain, no injury."

Finally, Rule 4 is to prevent injuries by using the correct exercise equipment. For example, wear a helmet for biking, eye guards for racquet ball, pads for roller blading, and of course, your parachute when sky diving. The correct footwear is important for most sports. It is often worth the extra expense to go to an athletic store where they know about shoes, and pay a little more for a good pair.

Looking like an athlete can also help. Some of us, who have the primitive gatherer gene, also have a need to shop. If you are in that group, brisk mall walking on a mission for the right sports clothes is an appropriate Preparation stage activity. Alternatively, if you are really self-confident and skilled at an activity, then a certain disdain for conforming with clothing norms can also work. It is a fine line, though.

While we were riding stationary cycles in the gym, a physician colleague and his young daughter came to exercise. Doctor dad was teaching her how to use a hula hoop. Still wearing his Elmer Fudd–type wool cap used by woodsmen in the great outdoors, he struggled to sustain more than two revolutions around his waist—something the seven-year-old did effortlessly. The dad, a respected brain surgeon, laughed for many minutes (so did we). As he continued to try the hula hoop, he ended up getting a great workout, despite how he looked. Clothes and skill level are only a small part of the whole story. Finding the fun in physical activity helps each of us stay the course to fitness and health.

Chapter 3

Exercise for Bone Health

Osteoporosis means porous bones—bones that gradually lose calcium, becoming less dense and more prone to breaking.

Lack of female or male hormones (estrogen and testosterone, respectively) increases your risk of osteoporosis.

Twenty-eight million Americans have osteoporosis, and more than 80 percent are women. Only a quarter of them know they have the problem, and only half of those are being treated. In the United States, osteoporosis costs $14 billion a year in health care.

"I think I'm shrinking," was Mary's reason for her clinic visit. At 64 years old, she was worrying about her bones. When she was 38, Mary had a hysterectomy for uterine cancer, and her ovaries were removed at the same time because estrogen hormones can stimulate the growth of uterine cancer cells. Despite her surgical menopause at a young age, Mary has never taken estrogen replacement therapy.

Mary tries to keep her bones strong by getting enough calcium and vitamin D. She does not smoke and rarely drinks alcohol, both of which can weaken bones. Physical activity strengthens bones, and Mary square dances two nights a week and walks most other days. She is in good health and looks forward to retiring in a few months. She plans on traveling and visiting her daughter's family in California.

Mary is a slender woman. She is 63 inches tall (she believes this is two inches less than her height in high school), and she weighs 118 pounds. Her general physical examination is normal. Studies were ordered to measure Mary's bone density.

Maybe because we see bones as a skeleton, we think of them as lifeless. Wrong! Bones are very much alive. Although two-thirds of a bone's weight is its calcified scaffolding, specialized bone cells make up the other one-third of its weight. The health and strength of our bones are tied closely to physical activity. When a bone is stressed, it becomes stronger. It is nature's way of reinforcing your bones. To build strong bones and keep them dense, you need to load, or stress, your bones with regular exercise.

The Importance of Strong Bones

At birth, our 270 bones lack calcium. As we grow, a bone's soft collagen framework rapidly stores calcium. Bones lengthen at special structures near their ends called *growth plates*. The growth plates allowed your bones to grow longer, while the rest of the bone remained strong to handle the forces you generated as an active youngster. When you reached your maximum height and linear growth stopped, the growth plates closed permanently. Some bones fuse together during growth, resulting in the 206 bones of the adult skeleton.

By the time you reach your twenties, you have achieved your *peak bone mass*. That is, your bones are as dense as they are ever going to be. Then, for your bones (as for many things), it is pretty much all downhill from there. But you can change the slope of that decline by the choices you make about diet and exercise.

Having strong, dense bones in your twenties is critical for preventing osteoporosis later in life. You can see the importance of your peak bone density in Figure 3.1. Bones get denser until your mid-twenties, then for the next 30 years, bone density does not change much. For women at the time of menopause, there are several years of a steep decline in bone density—up to 3 percent a year. That phase is followed by a more gradual decline, with losses of about 1 percent a year. A man's bone-loss curve looks similar, but the peak bone density is higher, and the decline in density is not as rapid as it is during menopause.

Your bones' activity does not end when you stop growing. Each year, about one-quarter of your skeleton is replaced. Two kinds of specialized bone cells, *osteoblasts* and *osteoclasts*, populate your bones' calcified scaffolding, and they are constantly remodeling your bones. The osteoclasts chew holes in your bones, while the osteoblasts lay down new bone. Without these cells to refurbish your bones, you could never heal a fracture. You can think of your bones as our highway system. Just when you think construction is finished, along comes a demolition team (the osteoclasts) tearing up the old road, followed closely by a construction crew (the osteoblasts) laying down a new one. Just as in road work, although day to day little appears to change, both crews are kept constantly busy.

When teenage boys use anabolic steroids, the high testosterone levels can trick their bones into thinking the boy is an adult man, which causes their growth plates to close prematurely. That is how anabolic steroids can stunt growth.

For most women in the United States, menopause occurs between the ages of 48 and 55, with the average being 51. Menopause can also be brought on instantly by surgical removal of the ovaries.

Men get osteoporosis too, but they are about 10 years behind women. That means a man of 70 has a bone density similar to a woman of 60.

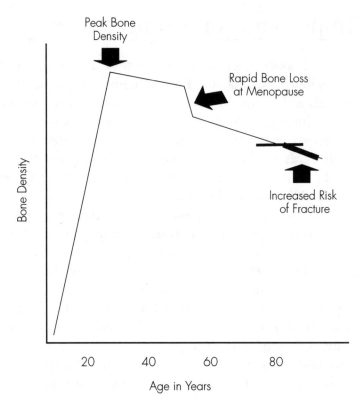

Figure 3.1   Bone density during a woman's lifetime.

Your Odds of Getting Osteoporosis

The balance between the forces of "good" and "evil" shown in Figure 3.2 determines whether you will have a net gain or loss in your bone density. The biggest factor affecting your bone density is your genetics. Seventy-five percent of your bone density is not under your control and results from your inheritance. How are your parents' and grandparents' bones? If they broke bones late in life or became stooped because of spinal compression fractures, you may be a prime candidate for osteoporosis.

Your race and frame size are two components of your inheritance that you can see. In general, Caucasians and Asians usually have weaker bones, while African-Americans' bones are more dense. Your body build also runs in the family, and slender, small-boned women

Studies suggest that getting enough calcium and getting regular exercise work together to build the strongest bones.

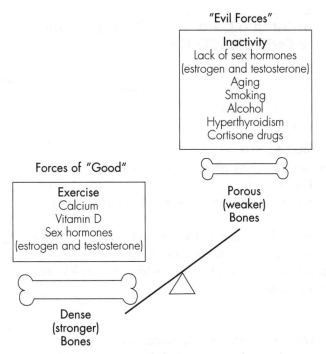

Figure 3.2 Forces that increase and decrease your bone density.

(those with petite frames) are at greatest risk for osteoporosis. Women can better gauge their risk for osteoporosis by completing the quiz in Table 3.1.

Prevention with Exercise and Calcium

The two factors over which you have the most control are your calcium intake and the amount of bone-loading exercise you get. Your peak bone mass is like your retirement fund, the nest egg that you will be living off later in life. (More accurately, the shell of the nest egg, as that is where eggs have all their calcium.) As an adult, your job is to preserve the nest egg.

To build up their accounts, growing adolescents need approximately 1,500 mg of calcium each day plus regular weight-bearing exercise. Unfortunately, we know from national surveys that the average

Smoking weakens your bones. Women who smoke have lower levels of estrogen and enter menopause at a younger age. Smoking may also reduce your ability to absorb calcium from your diet.

TABLE 3.1 Your Simple Calculated Osteoporosis Risk Estimate (SCORE)

	Your score

Add the points:
- If you are not African-American add 5 points   _____
- If you have rheumatoid arthritis add 4 points   _____
- If you have broken a bone with a minor injury after age 45, add 4 points for each fracture (maximum score 12)   _____
- If you have gone through menopause and have never received estrogen therapy add 1 point   _____
- Add 3 times the first digit of your age (for example, 74 years old = 7 × 3 = add 21) _____
- Divide your weight in pounds by 10 and round the result to the nearest whole number *for example, 163 pounds divided by 10 = 16.3, which rounds off to 16). Then, subtract your result from your score   –_____

   Your total score is   _____
If your total score is more than 5, you are at high risk for osteoporosis.

American gets only about 600 mg of calcium daily, and younger people, especially adolescent women, get even less than that. Also, the physical activity of young women markedly declines during their teenage years. Today, as inactive baby boomers approach old age, the combination of a longer life span, low calcium intake, and inactivity makes experts worry about a coming epidemic of osteoporosis.

An Ounce of Calcium is Worth a Pound of Fosamax[1]

From birth to old age, you need calcium for healthy bones. The recommended daily amount of calcium for different age groups is shown in Table 3.2. Many experts, such as those at the National Institutes of

---

[1] Fosamax is the trade name of alendronate, a drug used for the treatment of osteoporosis. It is discussed on page 46.

TABLE 3.2 **Recommended Calcium Intake**

	U.S. Recommended Daily Amount (RDA)	National Institutes of Health Recommendations
Children	800 mg	800 to 1,200 mg
Adolescents	1,200 mg	1,200 to 1,500 mg
Adults	800 mg	1,000 mg
Women after menopause	800 mg	If younger than 65 and HRT*: 1,000 mg If younger than 65, no HRT*: 1,500 mg If older than 65: 1,500 mg

*HRT is hormone or estrogen replacement therapy.

Health, feel the current recommended daily allowance (RDA) for calcium is too low, especially for the elderly. Table 3.3 lists the calcium content for different foods. You can see why if you do not like dairy products, it is difficult to get enough calcium without taking supplements. (How much broccoli can a person eat?)

Besides calcium, you need vitamin D for strong bones. Without vitamin D, children develop rickets. Vitamin D is found in foods such as

TABLE 3.3 **Calcium in Foods**

Food	Serving Size	Calcium per Serving	Calories per Serving
1% milk	1 cup	300 mg	120
1% cottage cheese	1/2 cup	100 mg	100
American cheese	1 slice	185 mg	70
Swiss cheese	1 slice	250 mg	70
Frozen yogurt	1/2 cup	100 mg	150
Yogurt	1 cup	300 mg	210
Fortified orange juice	8 ounces	240 mg	100
Sardines with bones	3 ounces	370 mg	200
Broccoli	1 cup	120 mg	30
Tofu	4 ounces	150 mg	170
Figs	10	250 mg	50

tuna, sardines, eggs, and fortified milk. Your skin can make vitamin D when it is exposed to sunlight's ultraviolet rays. Unfortunately, as you age, your skin is less able to make vitamin D. In addition, if you live north of 42 degrees, from November to February, there is not enough sunlight to make vitamin D, no matter what your age. In the United States, that would include half of Oregon and most of the states bordering Canada. In those regions, half of older individuals have low levels of vitamin D. Taking a once-a-day multivitamin will guard against a deficiency. Vitamin D is one of the fat-soluble vitamins, and it is stored in your body. Too much vitamin D can be harmful, so do not take additional vitamin D supplements without the advice of your health care provider.

The Results of Thin Bones

Osteoporosis means bones that are brittle and weakened from having less calcium and other minerals. By itself, osteoporosis does not cause any symptoms, which is why you cannot tell if you are developing it. The problem is that, as your bone density goes down, your chances of breaking a bone go up. Without measuring your bone density, you will learn about your weakened bones when you fall and your weakened femur (thigh bone) breaks, or you land on your outstretched arm and fracture bones in your forearm.

Measurement of bone density is useful for detecting osteoporosis, predicting your risk of a fracture, and monitoring your bone density.

Osteoporosis can also cause collapse of your back bones, or vertebrae (see Chapter 4, Figure 4.4 for a picture of your back bones). When these bones collapse, it can cause severe back pain that lasts weeks. For some unknown reason, at other times you do not feel the fracture. These spinal compression fractures are what cause women to lose height after menopause and develop a stooped posture, the so-called dowager's hump. (A dowager is an elderly woman with stately dignity and an elevated social status, often the widow of royalty. She was not someone who got much exercise.)

Losing more than two inches in height suggests that you have osteoporosis.

Detecting Osteoporosis

The way we usually look at bones is with an X ray. However, that is not a good way to learn about bone density. You have to lose one-third of a bone before the loss shows up on an X ray. In the last few years, new methods to measure bone density have been developed. These allow us to detect weakened bones long before they can be seen on an X ray. One method is called dual-energy X ray absorptiometry (DEXA). A DEXA scan takes only about 15 minutes and usually costs about $200. Although a DEXA scan uses radiation, it is only a tiny amount—about what you would get flying across the United States at 30,000 feet. A DEXA scan measures bone density in your spine and femur, or hip bone, two of the places where fractures from osteoporosis usually occur. Most times, if the density of those bones is low, your other bones will be less dense, too. The bone density in your arm or heel can be measured with a pDEXA (peripheral DEXA) scanner. Although these scanners are not as accurate in predicting your risk of breaking a bone, they are more portable, and the tests are less expensive.

In the summer of 1998, Medicare began paying for measurement of bone density when it is obtained to evaluate a postmenopausal woman's risk for osteoporosis and when it is used to monitor treatment of osteoporosis.

How Likely Are You to Break a Bone?

The results of a bone density measurement often are reported two ways: (1) how you compare with people of your age and sex (your *z-score*) and (2) how you compare with same-sex, younger individuals whose bone mass is at its highest level (your *t-score*). For each, your results show how many standard deviations your value is above or below the average. *Standard deviation* is a statistical term, and being one standard deviation below normal means that 65 percent of people have a value greater than yours. At two standard deviations below normal, your value is less than that of 95 percent of people. Translated into more meaningful words, your bone density decreases approximately 15 percent for each standard deviation. Losing only 15 percent of your bone density more than doubles your risk of a fracture.

Mary's spinal and femoral bone density *t-scores* were −4.5 and −3.1, respectively. That means her bone densities are only 40 and 55 percent of what is average for a young woman. Her laboratory studies showed normal blood levels of vitamin D, calcium, and thyroid hormone. Mary's family history, race, body build, and early menopause all worked against her bones.

Without exercise, her bone density would have been even worse. Physical activity always helps, but it might not be enough. If you have risks for osteoporosis (Figure 3.2), there may be reasons to measure your bone density, even if you get regular physical exercise.

Inactivity Is Bad for the Bones

Early anatomists noticed that bones were shaped by forces applied to them. Although we still do not know exactly how it works, bones respond to stress by becoming stronger. Without the stress, or loading, from physical activity, your bones lose calcium and become less dense. For example, your bones would lose calcium if you were confined to bed or the extreme inactivity of space flight. During weightlessness, bones lack even the usual forces of gravity. As a result, astronauts can lose 30 percent of their bone mass during a two-week space flight. Most times, your bones regain their original density when you get out of bed or splash down.

Elite junior weight lifters have bone densities that are 30 percent greater than those of non-weight-lifters of the same age. Resistance exercise, or weight training, probably most effectively stresses and builds your bones. Guidelines for strength training are presented in Chapter 12.

If exercise builds bones, then athletes should have denser bones than nonathletes. That is usually true. Skeptics might say that the difference in bone density is due to an athlete's better nutrition, lack of smoking, or some reason other than exercise. Luckily, tennis players are a natural experiment. By comparing a player's two arms, we can make sure that the only variable is exercise. Unlike the average person, elite tennis players have significantly more bone in their racquet arm than in their nondominant arm. Exercise made the difference. The findings show something else, too: the effects of physical activity are local—only the bones that are loaded get stronger.

Swimming will increase your endurance, but because it is a non-weight-bearing exercise, it is less effective than weight-bearing exercise for increasing bone density.

In 1996, researchers reviewed the world's literature about the kind of exercise it takes to strengthen our bones. They found two types of physical activity increase bone density. The first is strength, or weight, training. That makes sense because you put stress on your bones with every lift. Also, endurance activities such as running and gymnastics or games such as soccer, basketball, and volleyball increase bone mineral density. All are weight-bearing, or bone-loading, exercises: forces are applied to your spine and leg bones with the impact of each step.

What If You Already Have Osteoporosis?

Osteoporosis means your bones are more than 25 percent less dense than they should be. Once you have osteoporosis, you will always have weaker bones, but you can prevent further loss and even strengthen your bones. Regrettably, even the most effective therapy cannot increase your bone density back to a normal level. If you have osteoporosis, the first steps are getting enough calcium and vitamin D, plus additional tests to learn why your bones are weakened. Usually, bone loss is due to aging, your genetics, lack of sex hormones, or the other risks listed in Figure 3.2. Sometimes, certain medical disorders also contribute to the problem. Bones can be weakened by smoking, high thyroid hormone levels, particular medications (such as cortisone, Dilantin, and barbiturates), excessive alcohol intake, and a blood disorder called myeloma. These conditions are important to recognize, because specific treatment will be needed.

The World Health Organization defines osteoporosis as a bone density 2.5 standard deviations below the average of young normal individuals of your sex.

Exercise to Treat Osteoporosis

Exercise is an important part of your care if you have osteoporosis. You can benefit from (1) endurance and strength-training exercises, (2) learning posture and body movements that reduce your risk of injuring a bone, and (3) activities to prevent falls. In the first category, your goal is to use physical activity to strengthen your bones. Remember that weight-bearing endurance activities and strength-training exercises strengthen your bones best. Good choices for endurance activities are walking, stationary cycling, and water aerobics. For those with weakened bones, these activities avoid the excessive spinal loading of higher impact activities such as jogging or step aerobics. Endurance activities strengthen your leg muscles, and additional weight-training exercises can be gradually added to your workouts. Because of the potential for injury, begin weight lifting only after getting the advice of your health care provider. To make sure your technique and the lifts are appropriate, weight or strength training should be initiated with a physical therapist's supervision.

In just nine months, a group of women (average age 62 years) increased their bone density more than 5 percent with weight-bearing exercise that lasted 60 minutes, three times a week. A comparable group who did not exercise lost bone density.

If you have osteoporosis, avoid exercises that cause flexion of your trunk, such as abdominal crunches. These activities put too much stress on your spine.

Exercises that help maintain your posture and increase your stability while moving will reduce stress on your spine and decrease your chance of falling. Those activities include stretching your calf (Figure 12.11) and strengthening your thigh muscles. Your quadricep muscle (the front of your thigh) is strengthened by extending your leg while sitting (Figure 12.7). Moving your leg backward while standing (Figure 3.3) strengthens muscles on the back of your thigh. As you become stronger, an elastic band can be used to increase the resistance to your movements (Figure 3.4).

Having a rounded back (Figure 3.5) puts more stress on your vertebral bodies, increasing the risk of a compression fracture. Maintaining

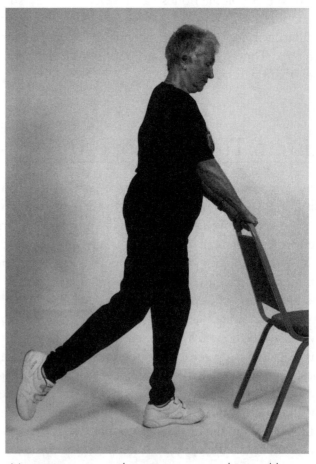

Figure 3.3   Movement to strengthen your posterior hip and leg muscles.

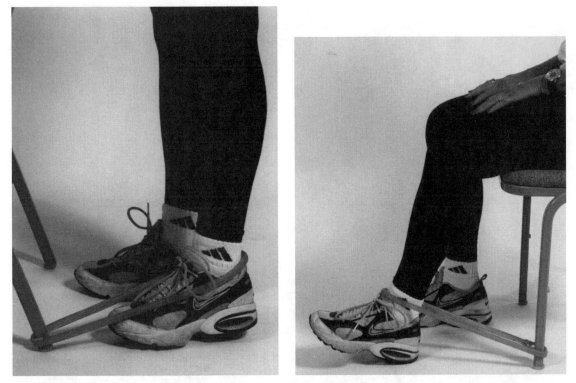

Figure 3.4   Elastic bands can be used to increase the resistance to leg movements.

the normal lordosis, or forward sway, in your lumbar spine (Figure 3.6) reduces the compression forces of your vertebral bodies.

If you fall, your risk of breaking a bone goes up as your bone density decreases. Besides strengthening your leg muscles, you can reduce your risk of falling by engaging in physical activities that improve your balance. The exercise Tai Chi has proven especially beneficial for improving balance. Tai Chi is a Chinese exercise that originated in the sixth century B.C. It is based on a set of 81 maneuvers, each done slowly, with one movement flowing gracefully into the next. In studies among the elderly, Tai Chi can increase fitness, coordination, balance, and body control. When studied, Tai Chi has been more effective than other physical activities for preventing falls. It is illustrated in Figure 3.7. The exercises can be learned from videotapes and books on Tai Chi. However, it is best learned in a class, where an insturctor can coach you on the movements.

Along with exercise, preventing falls involves fall-proofing your environment. That means, for example, no throw rugs, installing grab bars where needed, and wearing stabilizing shoes. It also means avoiding medications that can impair your thinking or coordination.

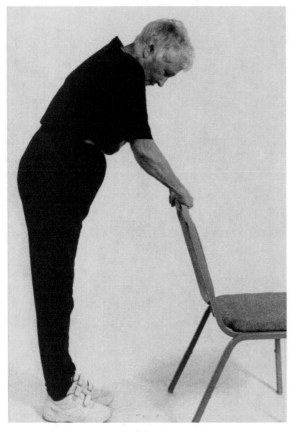

Figure 3.5   A rounded back puts more stress on your vertebral bodies.

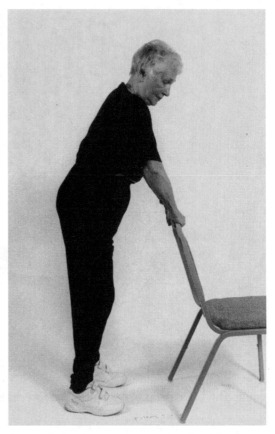

Figure 3.6   Stress on your vertebral bodies is decreased by bending your legs and maintaining the curve in your lower back.

Medications for Osteoporosis

Mary did not want to take any medications for her osteoporosis. She was willing to record her calcium intake and make sure she was getting at least 1,500 mg each day. After initial teaching from a physical therapist, Mary began using weight machines two or three times a week. Eighteen months after her initial assessment, Mary's bone density had increased 3 percent.

Medications are an option for the treatment of osteoporosis. If you are a woman who has stopped having periods, then estrogen replacement

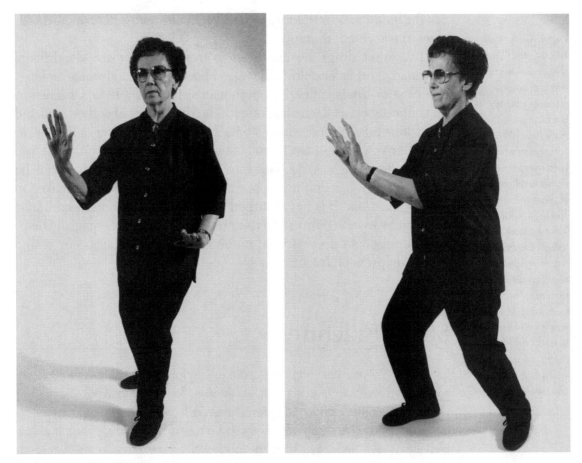

Figure 3.7   Tai Chi exercises.

therapy should be considered. This is especially true if you have re-
cently entered menopause, because that is the time when bone loss is
most rapid (Figure 3.1). Estrogen's ability to prevent bone loss is an
important factor to consider when you are weighing the risks and benefits of hormone replacement therapy. A major concern about estrogen
replacement therapy is its ability to stimulate breast tissue and poten-
tially increase a woman's risk of breast cancer. Raloxifene (Evista) is a
new "designer" estrogen and is a selective estrogen receptor modula-
tor. It is like estrogen in its protection of bones, but it does not stimulate breast tissue. (It also does not remedy hot flashes and may not
protect as well against heart disease.) For some women at increased

risk for breast cancer, raloxifene may be an alternative to standard hormone replacement therapy.

Two other drugs are approved to treat osteoporosis: alendronate (Fosamax) and calcitonin (Calcimar, Miacalcin). Alendronate belongs to a class of drugs called biphosphonates. It coats a bone's surface to prevent osteoclasts from attacking it. The drug is not absorbed well and so must be taken on an empty stomach, usually first thing in the morning. After you have taken it, you cannot go back to bed, either. If you did, the drug might slide back into your esophagus, where it can be very irritating. Calcitonin is a hormone your body normally makes to reduce bone loss. It is not absorbed at all from your stomach and must be given by injection or used as a nose spray. It may be especially helpful when used to decrease the immediate pain that can occur with a spinal compression fracture.

Stress Fractures

James is a 39-year-old man, with pain in his right foot. He is a recreational jogger and typically runs three miles, three or four times a week. About five weeks ago, James announced plans to run a marathon to commemorate his fortieth birthday. He had two months to train and began daily runs that doubled his weekly mileage. Then, he added two long runs on the weekend, and within a month, he had increased his training to approximately 40 miles a week. For the last 10 days, he has felt pain in his right foot. At first, aspirin lessened the discomfort, but soon, it became more painful. Now, just walking causes pain, and it aches even when he is in bed. James knew what he had done to himself by increasing his mileage so abruptly. His examination was notable for a sheepish look on his face and point tenderness along his fourth metatarsal (one of the five long bones in the foot).

Bone loading is important for building strong bones, but you can get too much of a good thing. When a bone is stressed, it is normal to experience microtrauma, which is microscopic damage to its structure. That microtrauma is expected and part of the bone strengthening process. After the microtrauma, the osteoclasts bone cells come in and clean up the problem. Then, the osteoblasts replace and reinforce the bone. The result is bone that is stronger than before. However, if the loading

The Women's Health Initiative study should give us answers to the effects of estrogen replacement therapy. It is a huge project with more than 100,000 participants who have been randomly assigned to different types of treatment—hormonal and nonhormonal—with systematic collection of outcomes regarding breast cancer, heart disease, osteoporosis, and mental functioning. Unfortunately, we will not know its results until 2005. For now, each woman must weigh the risks and benefits for herself.

Half of women and 20 percent of men over age 65 will have a fracture due to osteoporosis during their lifetime. Hip fractures can result in disability and death. A woman's risk of death from osteoporosis equals her risk of death from breast cancer.

is too frequent or intense, bone repair cannot keep up with the damage, and you get a stress fracture. Even strong, healthy bones can develop stress fractures when overloaded.

Breaking a bone usually happens suddenly because of an injury, but a stress fracture is different. It develops slowly. As a result, the discomfort of a stress fracture can wax and wane for weeks. Often, like James, you try to keep exercising, until the pain becomes too great to continue. The good news is that you often do not need to be in a cast when you have a stress fracture. Active rest is not just allowed, it is encouraged. That means you can alter your exercise and continue being physically active.

Stress fractures are so small that they may not show up on an X ray, and sometimes a bone scan or MRI (magnetic resonance imaging) scan is needed to show the fracture.

Continuing his training was not an issue for James. He was a long way from marathon condition, and he seemed relieved to have a reason to be excused from running his marathon. However, if he had wanted, he could have continued his jogging in a pool, supported by a flotation belt. After a few weeks of pool conditioning, he would be able to gradually resume jogging and slowly increase his mileage, especially during the next four to eight weeks, until his stress fracture's healing was complete.

Reasons for Stress Fractures

Stress fractures can have different causes. The first cause is an abrupt increase in training (as with James). The rule of thumb is that you should not boost your training more than 10 percent per week. Second, a stress fracture, like other overuse injuries, may be an indication of a mechanical problem. Perhaps, your stride is off or your technique is wrong, so forces are not being transmitted normally to your skeleton. It might be time to get some coaching or a gait analysis to correct a problem. Finally, a stress fracture can be a clue that you have osteoporosis. It might be a reason to measure your bone density and look for reasons why your bones are weakened.

Athletic Amenorrhea

Jenny did not look happy to be in the clinic. She was a junior in college and home for the summer. She came to the clinic reluctantly, at her mother's insistence. Jenny had not had a menstrual period for six months, and for the last three weeks her left foot had been hurting. Her mother was concerned that Jenny did not seem like her old self.

Jenny considered herself mildly obese until the summer after high school. That year, she worked as a life guard and lost 15 pounds by dieting and exercising daily. When she began college, she lost another 10 pounds, which she said was due to not liking the dorm food. She has weighed about the same since that time. Jenny said she eats three meals a day, but mainly fruits, salads, and popcorn.

At school, she was exercising in a physical education class three days a week, and most days she also ran four to six miles. Jenny said that her menses were regular until the last two years, when they became less frequent, occurring only three or four times each year. She had been sexually active in the past, but not for the last eight months.

Earlier this year, she noted pain and tenderness along the outside of her left foot. A podiatrist diagnosed a stress fracture. She had pain at one spot along her fifth metatarsal (the long bones between the ankle and toes), and an X ray showed a tiny break in the bone. Jenny switched to stationary cycling for four weeks, and her foot pain went away. She had been running again for a couple of months when the pain returned.

Jenny was 5 feet, 6 inches tall and weighed 120 pounds. Her body fat by skin-fold analysis was 14 percent (normal for women is 19 to 25 percent). Her general physical examination was normal, except for her low weight and tenderness at the midshaft of her left fourth metatarsal. Her bone density was 84 percent of what is average for a woman her age. Additional laboratory studies showed that Jenny did not have a reason for not having periods, other than excessive exercise combined with her low body weight.

Amenorrhea means missing three or more consecutive menstrual periods, and it can be caused by many medical conditions. A common reason is pregnancy. Having regular periods is linked to a woman's body weight. Until about age 10, boys and girls have similar body weights. Then, girls begin to gain body fat. They start having periods at about age 12, when their body fat has increased to 18 percent or more. If the percentage of fat later drops below this level, a woman's body senses that food is scarce and now is not the time to get pregnant. As a result, her brain stops making hormones to stimulate her ovaries. Her ovaries do not produce estrogen, her hormone levels fall, and menstrual periods stop. Just like the changes that occur at menopause, the reduced level of estrogen can weaken bones.

The normal body fat for women is approximately 23 percent.

Approximately 1 percent of adolescent girls develop anorexia nervosa. This dangerous disorder usually begins around the time of puberty and involves extreme weight loss—to at least 15 percent below the individual's normal body weight. Although these girls look emaciated, they are convinced they are overweight. With the weight loss, their periods stop. Sometimes they must be hospitalized to prevent starving to death.

Having a low body weight and missing menstrual periods can be clues to disordered eating. Eating disorders (anorexia and bulimia) are the third most common chronic illness among teenage women. Young women athletes are considered at especially high risk for disordered eating because social pressures toward thinness are made worse by influences from their sport. It is a popular notion that this problem is confined to gymnastics and ballet. Not true. At the middle and high school level, disordered eating behaviors are seen among young women from all sports. Eating disorders are serious conditions, and they have the highest mortality among all psychiatric diagnoses! People can develop severe metabolic abnormalities, muscle weakness, heart problems, and sudden death.

Despite exercising regularly, Jenny's bone density was less than expected, and she had another stress fracture in her foot. The reduced female hormone levels of athletic amenorrhea plus low calcium intake weaken bones. If young women like Jenny reduce their exercise and increase their intake of calories, they gain weight. With a higher weight (and higher percentage of body fat), a woman's hormone levels will increase, and she will restart normal menses. Although this type of bone loss may be reversible, its long-term effects are not known. In the short term, young athletes with weakened bones are at increased risk for stress fractures and scoliosis. They are also more likely to be injured.

Additional questioning revealed that Jenny had symptoms of depression. She was not sleeping well, felt she could not concentrate, and was not taking pleasure in anything. She had been using self-induced vomiting intermittently as a means to control her weight for a couple of years. She entered a counseling program, and over the next 16 months, her spirits and diet both improved. Her weight increased eight pounds, and her menses resumed. She experienced no further injuries.

Bottom Lines

Regular weight-bearing exercise is needed throughout your lifetime for bone health. Your bones reach their maximum density in your early twenties, and from then on, your bones gradually lose calcium. Several factors, in addition to exercise, slow that loss: adequate dietary calcium,

About 2 to 3 percent of young women develop bulimia nervosa. People with bulimia nervosa binge, or consume large amounts of food, and then purge their bodies of the excess calories by vomiting, abusing laxatives or diuretics, or exercising obsessively. In contrast to anorexia, those with bulimia may be normal or even a little overweight. Many individuals with bulimia, ashamed of their habits, do not seek help until they reach their thirties or forties. By this time, their eating behavior is deeply ingrained and more difficult to change.

In response to the growing problem of disordered eating, the American College of Sports Medicine published a position stand to alert people about the *female athlete triad*. Women with the triad have (1) disordered eating and use of physique-altering drugs (amphetamines, tobacco, anabolic steroids, diet pills, laxatives, and diuretics), and as a result, they get (2) amenorrhea and (3) osteoporosis.

Testosterone levels can decrease among men who exercise excessively, and analogous to women with amenorrhea, sport scientists have observed rare instances of athletic men with osteoporosis.

sufficient vitamin D, and normal levels of the sex hormones, estrogen and testosterone. As your bones become thinner and more porous, your chances of breaking a bone go up. Bone density can be measured to learn your risk of a fracture. The results may guide your subsequent care, and for women, influence the decision about taking hormone replacement therapy.

Stress fractures can be avoided by gradually increasing your exercise frequency and duration, and by cross training or alternating activities. Sometimes, a stress fracture will be an indication of an underlying problem in your bone health, such as occurs from the low-estrogen state found in eating disorders. Even with established osteoporosis, exercise is beneficial. However, because of a greater fracture risk, activities should be modified to gradually increase bone loading and minimize your chance of an injury.

Chapter 4

Exercise for Arthritis and Back Pain Relief

"I'm becoming the bionic woman," Lois said, and she was right. Having had both hips replaced and now facing knee surgery, she would be setting off metal detectors from three feet away. Lois had degenerative joint disease, also known as osteoarthritis, which is the most common form of arthritis.

Now 72 years old, Lois had always been an active person. When in her teens, she was an avid volleyball player and enjoyed hiking. She married in her twenties and had been a librarian, working part time when her children were small. Her husband was an art history professor, and most vacations were spent on trips, walking from galleries to old churches and other points of interest.

It was not until she was 50 that Lois first noticed pain in her groin when walking, and her X rays showed degenerative arthritis of her hip. Lois learned that her heredity was probably most responsible for her joint problem, and she was pleased when advised to stay active in spite of the joint damage. Lois was told that keeping muscles strong supports her joints and avoids a vicious cycle of inactivity, muscle weakness, less joint stability, more joint destruction, more pain, and even less activity.

Her left hip was replaced when she was 58, and the right hip about six years later. Now, her left knee had become so painful that she could not go beach walking to spot whales with her husband and grandchildren. She was anxious to proceed with knee replacement surgery and ready for the rehabilitation work that would follow. Being active helped Lois stay healthy—she was not overweight, had a normal blood pressure, and did not have diabetes, a high cholesterol level, or heart disease. Her risk from surgery was low, despite her age.

Arthritis means joint inflamation. *Rheumatism* is a more general term that refers to pain or other symptoms anywhere in your musculoskeletal system. More than 100 different problems can cause pain in your joints.

One in seven Americans has arthritis. The most common types are osteoarthritis (20.7 million adults), fibromyalgia (3.7 million adults), rheumatoid arthritis (2.1 million adults), and gout (2.1 million adults).

Wear-and-Tear Osteoarthritis

The most common type of arthritis is osteoarthritis, also called degenerative joint disease or wear-and-tear arthritis. The bony surfaces of your joints are covered with cartilage. Cartilage is made of specialized cells, and it forms the shiny smooth tissue that lubricates joints and cushions their surface. With aging, cartilage thins, stiffens, and becomes frayed. When your car's brake pads are worn, you can replace them, but you cannot replace your joint surfaces. Once the cartilage is worn, it does not regenerate. Without it, bone rubs on bone, and that causes pain.

It is not known why some peoples' joints wear out faster than others.

Also, with less cartilage as a shock absorber, more stress is placed on the underlying bone. This causes the bone to form overgrowths around the joint. If you look at the hands of many people in their seventies, you can see that their finger joints closest to their fingertips are enlarged. The enlargement is due to worn cartilage and growth of bone around the joint. (Despite what you might have heard, osteoarthritis of your fingers is not from cracking your knuckles.)

Osteoarthritis primarily affects older adults. The older you are, the more likely you are to have degenerative joint disease. Only about 2 percent of those younger than age 45 have osteoarthritis, whereas by the time we are 65, more than two-thirds will have it. The joints usually affected by osteoarthritis are in your hands and the weight-bearing joints in your legs.

Capsaicin is a cream made from pepper juice and available without a prescription. It causes pain fibers to release all their chemical transmitters, and once these cells are depleted, you no longer feel pain. It must be used several times a day to be effective.

Osteoarthritis of the hands and hips tends to run in families, but some conditions increase your risk. For example, a hip that has been abnormal since birth, or a previously damaged knee joint would predispose you to developing osteoarthritis, as do being overweight and having diabetes or gout. The medications used to treat osteoarthritis are pain relievers such as acetaminophen, nonsteroidal anti-inflammatory drugs (NSAIDs, pronounced "N-saids") such as ibuprofen and naprosyn, and topical capsaicin.

Will Exercise Cause My Joints to Wear Out Faster?

Arthritis researchers (and many of the rest of us) have worried about whether exercise might speed the process of joint damage. It is not an easy question to answer. To know for sure, you would like to assign young people to either regular exercise or no exercise, and then see what happens to their joints over the next 50 years. Even if physical activity speeds joint wear, it would take many years to see a difference between the two groups. Keeping the experiment going long enough to get an answer would be impossible. Instead, scientists studied those already in their sixties and seventies. They asked those people about their exercise habits and measured joint damage by physical examination and X rays. Contrary to what you might think, people who exercised had no more arthritis than nonexercisers. In putting together all the evidence gathered so far, the bottom line is that exercise will not wear out your joints prematurely. Exercise does not damage joints. In fact, even if you already have arthritis, your joints *benefit* from regular physical activity. Joint movement helps keep cartilage healthy by stimulating it to take up nutrients and dispose of waste products. In addition, exercise strengthens muscles so that they can better support your joints.

Can Exercise Help Osteoarthritis?

Exercise can help joints damaged from arthritis. In 1997, researchers reported results of an 18-month-long study of exercise for knee degenerative arthritis. More than 400 people participated. All were older than age 60 and already had knee damage from osteoarthritis as determined by X rays. They were assigned to one of three groups: (1) those who followed a regular walking program, (2) those who did leg-strengthening exercises, or (3) a control group who did not exercise. They found that after one-and-a-half years of regular physical activity, both exercise groups had less knee pain and fewer physical limitations due to their arthritis than those who did not exercise. The exercisers also increased their ability to walk distances and climb stairs. Their improvement was not just due to exercisers getting used to their knee discomfort, because despite their regular exercise, X rays showed that those participants had no worsening of their knee arthritis.

If you have osteoarthritis, before beginning regular exercise, it is useful to get advice from your health care provider about your body mechanics and answers to the following questions. *Would your joint problem be helped by specific exercises to strengthen muscles around the joint?* For example, chronic knee pain can result from your patella

COX-2 inhibitors are a new type of non-steroidal anti-inflammatory drug that are specific for inhibiting cyclooxygenase (the COX enzyme) at sites of inflammation. They avoid adverse effects on enzyme systems in your stomach and the resultant gastrointestinal side effects. In 1999, Celecoxib (Celebrex) and rofecoxib (Vioxx) were approved for relief of the signs and symptoms of osteoarthritis and rheumatoid arthritis. Studies are underway to better define the benefits and risks of this new class of drugs.

Rather than being harmful, exercise is good for your joints, even if you already have arthritis. Now, we know that exercise is part of the treatment for degenerative joint disease.

Glucosamine sulfate (1,500 mg per day) and chondroitin sulfate (1,200 mg per day) are nutritional supplements reported in short-term studies to be effective in treatment of osteo-arthritis. Over several weeks, they appear to have beneficial effects on joint cartilage metabolism and also may be weakly anti-inflammatory.

(knee cap) not moving in its normal groove when you bend and straighten your leg. This misalignment wears cartilage off the underside of your knee cap, leading to osteoarthritis. If that is your problem, then doing specific exercises can strengthen your medial quadriceps (the inner portion of your thigh muscle) to help the patella stay on track.

Would a brace, elastic support, or taping be helpful? Perhaps you had a badly sprained ankle a couple of years ago. Although healed, your ankle is a little stiff and seems prone to being resprained. Your ankles (and other joints) have specialized sensory nerves that provide your body with information about the joint's position. Those nerves can be damaged when your ankle is injured. As a result, your ankle will never be quite as good at letting you know its position, and you won't be as effective in making adjustments to avoid an injury. A lace-up ankle brace can help stabilize the joint. Also, your skin rubbing on the brace is another source of feedback to your body about your ankle's position.

Are there mechanical problems to be corrected? If you have an injury or arthritis, you know that your body tries to compensate. If you have arthritis of your ankle, you might compensate by altering your natural gait—locking your ankle in one position and running more on your forefoot. By changing your stride, your gait's natural symmetry is lost. Before long, your back starts aching. Sometimes, in addition to worrying about an injured joint, compensatory mechanical habits need to be corrected to avoid future problems.

Although exercising a damaged joint might not wear it out faster, it sometimes causes pain and stirs up inflammation. This can be kept to a minimum by taking two aspirins or a nonsteroidal anti-inflammatory drug (NSAID) before exercise and icing the joint immediately after finishing your workout. If joint pain lasts more than two hours after exercise or is getting worse with each workout, check with your health care provider. Table 4.1 lists additional tips for exercising with osteoarthritis.

TABLE 4.1 **Tips for Exercising with Osteoarthritis**

- Choose exercises that minimize joint stress and strengthen muscles around arthritic joints.
- Seek advice about specific exercises to stabilize joints and correct any mechanical problems.
- Ask whether a brace, elastic wrap, or taping would be helpful.
- Consider taking aspirin or a nonsteroidal anti-inflammatory drug (NSAID) before exercise and icing a joint immediately after your workout.
- Warm up your muscles and joints before exercise and use gentle stretches to increase joint flexibility.

After her surgery, it took Lois quite a while to feel steady when walking, and she began using a cane. Her unsteadiness was partly because joints have specialized nerve cells that tell the body the joint's position. You lose those nerves when a joint is replaced. Although Lois's stability has returned, a tall carved walking stick has become a companion on her frequent strolls.

Arthritis, Tendinitis, and Bursitis

Itis means inflamed. So, *arthritis* is an inflamed joint, *tendinitis* is an inflamed tendon, and *bursitis* is an inflamed bursa. Tendons are the grisly tissue that attach muscle to bone. Ligaments connect bone to bone. Bursas are places that lubricate where tendons or ligaments run by each other. Just like a joint, these structures can become inflamed. *Rheumatism* and *rheumatic disorders* are general terms for inflamation anywhere in the musculoskeletal system. Figure 4.1 shows common sites of *itis* that do not involve a joint.

> Choose an activity that minimizes the trauma to your joints and strengthens the supporting muscles. Avoid jarring impacts, for example, jumping off your board in step aerobics. Walking has one-third the lower extremity joint stress of jogging. Non-weight-bearing exercise using a stationary cycle further reduces the stress on your hips, knees, and ankles.

Orin is a 32-year-old man who works for the home office of a college fraternity. His job frequently requires him to travel, and Orin has become familiar with the concourses in the major hub airports. He has raced through most of them trying to make connections.

Orin's joint problems began when he played football for the winning team of a small Division III liberal arts college. Late in the season of his senior year, he thought he had twisted his right knee, but the injury was slow to heal. Orin's knee remained warm and swollen. In the mornings, it was stiff, and it took him over an hour to loosen it up. Despite the end of the season and trials of different nonsteroidal anti-inflammatory drugs (NSAIDs), his knee did not improve. Orin was finally sent to an arthritis specialist.

The rheumatologist (a physician who specializes in arthritis) learned that Orin also had back stiffness in the mornings. X rays of Orin's back and blood tests showed that the problem was more than a football injury. Orin had a type of inflammatory arthritis called ankylosing spondylitis.

Arthritis can be divided into two broad categories: inflammatory and noninflammatory. Table 4.2 lists examples of both types and their characteristics. Deciding which of these you have narrows down what is causing your joint pain. And as you might expect, anti-inflammatory drugs are most useful for inflammatory arthritis. Both NSAIDs and

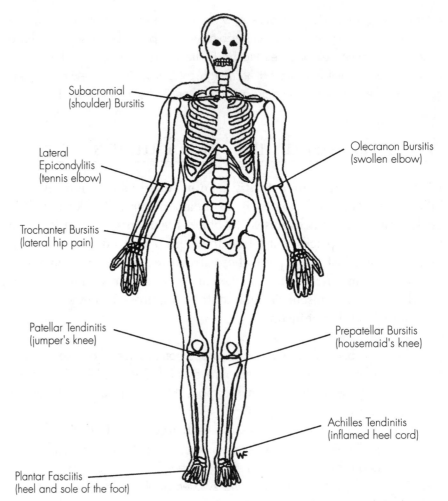

Subacromial
(shoulder) Bursitis

Olecranon Bursitis
(swollen elbow)

Lateral
Epicondylitis
(tennis elbow)

Trochanter Bursitis
(lateral hip pain)

Patellar Tendinitis
(jumper's knee)

Prepatellar Bursitis
(housemaid's knee)

Achilles Tendinitis
(inflamed heel cord)

Plantar Fasciitis
(heel and sole of the foot)

Figure 4.1   The most common sites for inflammation (bursitis and tendinitis) that do not involve a joint.

Most people with anky-losing spondylitis de-velop the problem before age 40. Men are affected with the disorder five times more than women.

aspirin also relieve pain, and that is the primary reason that they are used for noninflammatory arthritis.

Degenerative joint disease, the most common arthritis, is non-inflammatory. Orin's symptoms and examination suggested inflammatory arthritis and a condition called ankylosing spondylitis. The word *anky-losing* has a Greek origin and means bent and stiffened. *Spondylitis* is inflammation of the spine. The hallmark of ankylosing spondylitis is inflammation leading to stiffening of the spine and sacroiliac joints (where your spine attaches to your pelvis).

TABLE 4.2   **Inflammatory versus Noninflammatory Arthritis**

	Inflammatory	**Noninflammatory**
Kinds of arthritis	Rheumatoid arthritis, lupus erythematosis, ankylosing spondylitis, gout, and joint infections	Osteoarthritis, trauma, mechanical problems or loose body in the joint, and avascular necrosis
How did the problem start?	Can begin with gradual stiffening of joints but is often more rapid in onset; arthritis severity can fluctuate, with times of more and less inflammation	Onset of osteoarthritis usually after age 40; often chronic, with gradual worsening
What happens with rest and activity?	Joint pain can occur at rest; joints stiffen when inactive, and that stiffness can take more than one hour to loosen up (prolonged morning stiffness)	Joint pain often worse with use and better with inactivity; stiff joints loosen up faster (less than 30 minutes of morning stiffness)
What do the involved joints look like?	Joints are painful, warm, reddened, and swollen with extra joint fluid; it is the inflammation that causes joints to be "on fire" or "in flames"; joints are tender when touched and with movement	Often affects weight-bearing joints; possible history of recent or prior joint injury; joints can be tender, but with less warmth and swelling than in inflammatory arthritis
How do the joints end up?	Joint inflammation also can involve tendons and ligaments around the joint; with chronic inflammation, joint deformities and destruction can occur (crippling arthritis)	Tendons and ligaments around the joint usually not involved; joints are stiff and have less motion than normal; a grating (crepitus) can be heard or felt with joint movement

Have you seen an older man, stooped over and walking stiffly, with his head not moving to either side? He probably has ankylosing spondylitis. The joints between the back bones are inflamed (see page 67 for a discussion of backbone anatomy). The joints stiffen and give a characteristic appearance on an X ray. After many years, the inflammation causes the individual vertebrae to lose joint motion and become completely fused. At that point, the back is no longer painful. However, because it is stiffened, the spine loses its ability to absorb a shock and is more prone to spinal fractures.

The shoulders, leg joints, and tendons can also be affected. Rarely, the inflammation involves other parts of the body, such as the eye, heart, and lungs. Ankylosing spondylitis tends to run in families. For

Gout typically occurs among men over age 45. Severe joint pain develops suddenly, and the affected joint becomes tender, warm, and swollen. Uric acid, normally present in your blood and joint fluid, crystalizes out in the cooler joints of your feet (most commonly the joint at the base of your big toe). The crystals cause joint inflamation. Gout can be prevented by lowering uric acid levels. Once gout is under control, people can exercise normally.

NSAIDs all work in similar ways to decrease inflammation. Examples of these drugs are diclofenac (Voltaren, Cataflam), etodolac (Lodine), ibuprofen (Motrin, Advil, Nuprin), indomethacin (Indocin), ketoprofen (Orudis), meclofenamate (Meclomen), naproxen (Aleve, Naprosyn, Anaprox), piroxicam (Feldene), sulindac (Clinoril), and tolmetin (Tolectin). They all have similar side effects, too. They can cause bleeding from your stomach, high blood pressure, fluid retention, and kidney damage.

unknown reasons, people can vary greatly in the problems they have from this condition. Some live their whole lives with only mild low back pain, whereas others have many problems beginning at a young age, including the need for joint replacements and back surgery.

Joint inflammation with ankylosing spondylitis is usually treated with NSAIDs. Occasionally, injecting corticosteroids (cortisone) into involved joints, muscle relaxants, and low-dose oral cortisone are used as additional therapy. Immunosuppressive drugs (such as methotrexate and gold salts) that can benefit other types of inflammatory arthritis are not very helpful for ankylosing spondylitis. Exercise, to maintain spinal flexibility and proper joint alignment, is a critical part of treatment.

Orin was given indomethacin, which is an NSAID. It often is better than other drugs for reducing inflammation but is also harder on the stomach and more likely to cause stomach ulcers and bleeding. Although not usually used long term, it can be helpful to get inflammation under control. Orin's knee swelling slowly improved, and it has not bothered him again. Being an athlete, he knew the importance of conditioning and was used to training. This time, a physical therapist was the coach, and the drills were exercises to keep his spine flexible. Although he still has morning back stiffness, it is well controlled with a dinnertime NSAID. He is religious about his flexibility program and adds swimming three or four times a week. Swimming is an excellent exercise for Orin. It limits joint trauma, gives him cardiovascular endurance, and helps his back, shoulders, and hips remain limber.

Rheumatoid Arthritis

Bud wondered what was causing his foot pain. His aching feet made him feel older than his 34 years. Although he had not changed his activities, each morning Bud awoke with stiff and painful feet. Usually, things were better after a hot shower. He tried buying new shoes and added a gel shoe insert, without much improvement.

Bud had wrestled in high school and played intramural sports in college. He had his share of sore shoulders and knees, but no major joint injuries. Bud was an assistant pastor at a large local church, and he enjoyed tennis and hiking with his young family. Prior to his aching feet, Bud felt healthy and had not seen a doctor in years.

Bud's feet had been hurting for several weeks by the time he finally came into the clinic. His morning stiffness had spread to involve his wrists and left knee. Bud's physical examination showed thickening of the joint lining of his wrists, ankles, and knee. Those joints were warm, tender, and had less flexibility than normal joints. In addition, he had hard, small lumps along the outside surface of his forearms. (These were rheumatoid nodules, which can occur with rheumatoid arthritis.) His blood tests and wrist and feet X rays showed changes characteristic of rheumatoid arthritis.

Bud grew up in Wisconsin, where he hiked, camped, and canoed most summers. Bud and his doctors wondered whether his arthritis could be caused by Lyme disease, which is found in that area.

Rheumatoid arthritis is the most common inflammatory arthritis. People of all races have rheumatoid arthritis, and women are affected three times more often than men. The problem often comes on gradually. In the early stages, you might have only sore, stiff hands or feet when awakening or sitting for more than 30 minutes. As the disease progresses, joints become red, swollen, and tender. The joint inflammation can involve tissues around joints. It is destruction of the tendons and ligaments around joints that causes them to develop the deformities of crippling arthritis.

As with most inflammatory arthritis, the disease can involve other body parts. The same type of inflammation that affects a joint can occur in the outside lining of the eye, parts of the lung, or the covering of the heart. Drugs are used to both decrease inflammation (NSAIDs and occasionally corticosteroid pills) and prevent further changes (drugs to suppress the immune system, such as gold therapy and methotrexate). The criteria used to diagnose rheumatoid arthritis are shown in Table 4.3.

Can Exercise Help Inflammatory Arthritis?

In the past, people with inflammatory arthritis were advised to rest when their joints were painful. Although their inactivity reduced joint inflammation, it weakened their muscles. In addition, their joints stiffened and

Some rheumatic diseases are difficult to diagnose. Even among people with the same condition, how the illness starts, which joints are inflamed, and what other tissues are involved can differ. Because the illnesses can be so variable, expert panels have been assembled to agree on criteria for many rheumatic disorders.

In 1976, Lyme disease was recognized as an illness. It is caused by the bacterium *Borrelia burgdorferi,* which is carried by the deer tick. You become infected from these ticks. The disease's initial and most distinctive feature is a patch of red rash that starts at the site of the tick bite. That rash occurs in 75 percent of those with Lyme disease. Soon after the bite, a person can have general complaints such as fever and chills. If the illness is not treated, weeks to months following the bite, a relapsing inflammatory arthritis of the knees, shoulders, elbows, ankles, or wrists can develop. Approximately 10 percent of people with Lyme disease will also have problems with their nervous system or heart.

TABLE 4.3   **Is It Rheumatoid Arthritis?**

Rheumatoid arthritis is definitely present if you have four or more of these findings:

- Swelling in three or more joint areas for at least six weeks
- Joint involvement that is similar on both sides of your body
- Involvement of hand joints and wrists for six weeks or longer
- More than one hour of joint stiffness when you wake up
- Rheumatoid nodules (bumps along the undersurface of your forearms)
- Positive blood test for rheumatoid factor
- Specific changes seen on X rays of your hands or wrists
- X rays showing thinning of the bone next to an inflamed joint

Other findings can include weight loss, low-grade fever, eye inflammation, dry eyes and mouth, inflammation of the outside lining of the heart (pericarditis) and lungs (pleuritis), enlarged spleen, and frequent infections.

Because rheumatoid arthritis can involve the heart, lungs, and cervical spine (neck), it is important to see your health care provider before beginning regular exercise. Also, rheumatoid arthritis frequently affects your feet, and expertly fitted shoes can be especially important.

By *exercise*, we do not mean just gentle stretching. In fact, when flexibility exercises were compared with cycling and brisk walking, the more intense activities resulted in the greatest improvements. Even when followed for a decade, people with rheumatoid arthritis who exercised did not have more inflamed or damaged joints.

became less flexible. Better understanding of inflammatory arthritis led to a complete turnaround in what is recommended.

Exercise scientists found that people advised to rest their inflamed joints were given a double whammy against their ability to move. First, when joints are stiff and sore, the metabolic cost of movement is increased about 50 percent. That is, to do the same activity with inflammatory arthritis, you need to be in better shape. Secondly, when advised to rest, people with rheumatoid arthritis get deconditioned, and their stamina and strength are reduced. People with rheumatoid arthritis needed more muscle power, but by resting their joints, they ended up with less.

It was not until the 1970s that Swedish doctors questioned the wisdom of rest as a treatment for rheumatoid arthritis and began studying exercise for patients with inflamed joints. Researchers found (you guessed it) that regular physical activity was beneficial. Now, exercise is part of the treatment for inflammatory arthritis. Rather than being harmful, exercise reduces joint destruction. Importantly, people with rheumatoid arthritis who exercise are able to be more active and have fewer limitations as a result of their joint problems.

As a person with inflammatory arthritis, when you begin a program of physical activity, you should work on (1) cardiovascular endurance, (2) muscle strength, and (3) joint flexibility. Additional tips for exercising with inflammatory arthritis are listed in Table 4.4.

Your endurance is increased with aerobic conditioning, which requires sustained activity of your large muscle groups, such as occurs

---

TABLE 4.4 **Tips for Exercising with Inflammatory Arthritis**

- Get medical clearance, especially if your illness affects your heart, lungs, or neck.
- Select low-impact aerobic exercises that will not stress your joints (such as swimming, cycling, or walking).
- Warm up your muscles and joints before exercise and use gentle stretches to increase joint flexibility.
- Gradually increase the duration of exercise until you can train for 45 minutes four days a week.
- Seek advice about specific strengthening exercises, braces, or elastic wraps to stabilize involved joints and correct any mechanical problems.
- Seek medical advice if any joint suddenly becomes more inflamed or pain lasts more than two hours after exercise.

---

with walking, swimming, or cycling. To avoid injury and maximize your training benefits, instruction on flexibility and strengthening exercises from a physical therapist is often helpful. Examples of flexibility exercises are illustrated in Figures 12.11 and 12.12 (calf), A.6 and A.7 (wrist), and 12.13 and 12.14 (shoulder). Flexibility of your neck can be aided by slowly moving your head forward and backward (Figure 4.2) eight times.

Bud had none of the other problems that are sometimes seen with Lyme disease. However, the rheumatologist recommended a course of antibiotics on the remote chance that Lyme disease was causing Bud's arthritis. Bud took antibiotics for several weeks, without an effect on his symptoms or joint inflammation.

Bud wanted to begin exercising. To help him with specific advice for training, he underwent an exercise test in the Human Performance Laboratory. He was not able to go very far on the treadmill, but his problem was not with his heart or his lungs. He was limited by his muscles, which placed him in the low fitness category. Bud did not realize how much he had limited his physical activities and how out of shape he was. Bud began with a month of twice-weekly physical therapy to learn specific exercises and correct gait changes that were caused by his arthritis. He had special shoes made that were well cushioned and supported his feet.

For the first two months, Bud did warm-water aerobics at the local YMCA. As his fitness improved and his joint inflammation lessened, he started power walking and jogging on a padded track. He joined a local gym to lift weights and use a stationary exercycle. Although Bud takes daily medication and still has some joint stiffness, he has no physical limitations and continues to do well.

If you have arthritis, exercise in a warm-water pool (83°F to 87°F). The warmth increases your flexibility, and the water reduces joint stress. The YMCA and the Arthritis Foundation have designed water exercise programs for people with arthritis. Check with your local pools about warm-water exercise.

People who have taken corticosteroids (prednisone or cortisone) can develop a problem with their hip and shoulder joints called avascular necrosis. The bone near the joint does not get enough blood flow and breaks down. If you have taken cortisone and have joint pain, see your health care provider before starting to exercise.

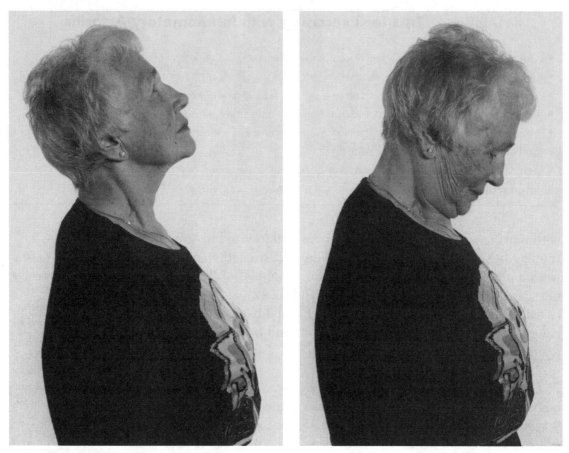

Figure 4.2   Stretches for neck flexibility.

Other Types of Inflammatory Arthritis

Following a cortico-steroid injection, a joint needs to be rested. Ask your health care provider for advice about how to modify your activity immediately after a joint injection.

Other illnesses can cause inflammatory arthritis, such as systemic lupus erythematosis and scleroderma. These disorders are sometimes called autoimmune disorders because the body seems to make antibodies against itself. Tables 4.5 and 4.6 list the criteria used to identify lupus erythematosis and scleroderma. Less is known about exercise with these disorders. However, the general recommendations are similar to the advice for people with rheumatoid arthritis. Because of potential problems that affect your ability to exercise (such as high blood pressure, heart problems, and muscle inflammation), see your health care provider before beginning regular physical activity.

TABLE 4.5   Is It Systemic Lupus Erythematosis?

Four of the following are needed for the diagnosis:

- Skin rash on the upper cheeks
- Skin rash caused by sunlight
- Sores in the mouth
- Seizures or mental illness
- Joint pain and swelling, but usually not the joint deformities seen with rheumatoid arthritis
- Inflammation of the outside lining of the heart or lungs
- Kidney damage
- Abnormalities in the blood count
- Positive ANA (antinuclear antibody) blood test
- Other positive blood tests for lupus antibodies

Fibromyalgia

Alice did not want to see another physician about her muscle pains. She had already been told by several doctors that nothing was wrong. Still, she was sure it wasn't all in her head. Alice had been well until about two years ago. At that time, after a particularly nasty case of the flu, her fatigue and muscle pains never seemed to go away. Several months later, she saw her primary care doctor, who took some blood tests and X rays. The results were normal, and although that was reassuring, Alice did not feel any better.

As the weeks dragged on, Alice also saw a psychologist. Because depression can cause fatigue and physical complaints, Alice's doctor thought a

---

TABLE 4.6   Is It Scleroderma?

Affected individuals have symmetric skin thickening of their hands, arms, or face and two of the following:

- Sclerodactyly (skin changes limited to the fingers)
- Ulcers at the tips of the fingers
- Lung disease seen on chest X ray

Other findings can include a history of Raynaud's phenomenon (fingers turn white, blue, then red, when exposed to the cold), heart damage, muscle inflammation, gastrointestinal problems, high blood pressure, and kidney damage.

Often, it is hard to tell which came first—feeling sad and having the aches and pains that can go with depression, or having aches and pains and then feeling sad about not being well.

counselor could help in deciding whether Alice was depressed. However, the psychologist and a trial of antidepressant medication both indicated that depression was not Alice's problem.

Because of her muscle pains, Alice was referred to a neurologist, who ordered muscle enzyme studies and electrical tests of her muscles. Those results were normal, too. Finally, Alice was referred to our Human Performance Laboratory for testing, to see if she had a problem with muscle metabolism. She looked like a healthy 30-year-old woman, and it was easy to see why she had been mistakenly told that nothing was wrong. However, when examined, Alice had all the findings of fibromyalgia.

Fibromyalgia follows osteoarthritis as the second leading cause of muscle and joint problems. It also is referred to as the fibromyalgia syndrome or fibrositis. Although fibromyalgia is a rheumatic disorder, there is no arthritis. Fibromyalgia strikes your soft tissues, resulting in muscle aches and pains. Because those affected are usually young women (85 percent of those with fibromyalgia are female) with many symptoms and few physical examination abnormalities, they are often thought of as complainers.

Today, it is recognized that people with fibromyalgia have distinct physical examination findings. The disorder is diagnosed when you have more than three months of muscle pain and tenderness when pressure is applied to specific trigger points (listed in Table 4.7 and shown in Figure 4.3). The remainder of the physical examination often is normal. In addition, sufferers of fibromyalgia have a sleep disturbance and do not have enough REM or deep restorative sleep, resulting in feeling unrested and chronically tired. Occasionally, fibromyalgia seems to be brought on by something specific—an infection, an automobile accident, or another illness. However, most times, it comes on gradually. If you have fibromyalgia, you have some good days, some not so good days, and some really bad days. Symptoms can be worsened by stress, damp and cold weather, and vigorous or jarring exercise.

What Causes Fibromyalgia?

No one knows what causes fibromyalgia. Its treatment is aimed at reducing symptoms. Many are relieved just to have their complaints diagnosed and learn that it is not "just in my head." Medications are sometimes used to correct the disordered sleep, including low-dose amitryptyline (Elavil), cyclobenzaprine (Flexeril), doxepin, paroxetine

---

TABLE 4.7   **Is It Fibromyalgia?**

Fibromyalgia is diagnosed when you have the following:

- Fatigue and widespread muscle pain for more than three months
- 11 of 18 trigger points are painful*
    - Occiput (base of the skull) (both sides)
    - Upper fold trapezius (upper back) (both sides)
    - Lateral epicondyle (outer side elbow) (both sides)
    - Supraspinatus (inner side of the shoulder blade) (both sides)
    - Second costochondral junction (junction rib and breast bone) (both sides)
    - Upper outer buttocks (both sides)
    - Greater trochanter (outer side of the hip) (both sides)
    - Fat pad inside of the knee (both sides)
    - Lumbar spine (low back)
    - Posterior low cervical spine (lower neck)

*Trigger points are checked with the examiner's thumb, using enough pressure to blanch the thumbnail. This pressure produces more pain (not just tenderness) at trigger points than at other sites.

(Paxil), nefazodone (Serzone), and clonazepam (Klonopin). The muscle aches can be helped by NSAIDs, capsaicin, massage, acupuncture, and a gradual low-impact exercise program.

Can Exercise Help Fibromyalgia?

We and others at our hospital are interested in fibromyalgia. People with fibromyalgia feel fatigued, even with very little exertion, and their muscles often hurt after exercise. This made physiologists wonder whether people with fibromyalgia have problems with how their muscles metabolize fuel. Studies show that their muscle metabolism is normal, but those with fibromyalgia tend to be very deconditioned. If you have fibromyalgia, you can benefit from exercise. When trained with gradual low-intensity aerobic conditioning, your fitness will increase, and muscle pain and fatigue will be less.

Begin with only five minutes of exercise and add two minutes every three days. Try to work up to 45 minutes of continuous activity most days of the week.

With fibromyalgia, you will want to choose exercises that are low intensity and do not jolt your muscles and joints. For example, step aerobics would be a mistake because of its pounding of your joints and muscles. Walking, swimming, or stationary cycling are good choices.

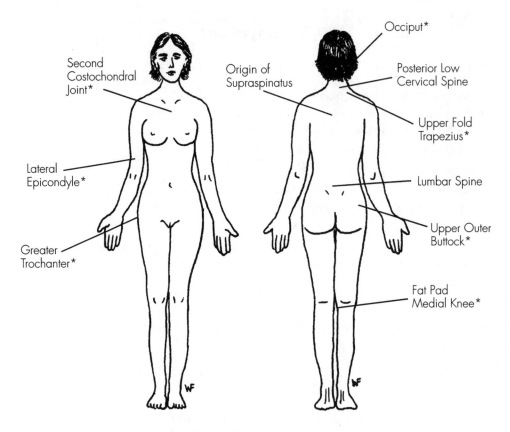

*Trigger points on both sides of the body

Figure 4.3   Fibromyalgia is characterized by tenderness of at least eleven of these eighteen specific locations.

Those with fibromyalgia are also prone to developing delayed muscle soreness, which is pain that comes on a day or two after exercise. If this occurs, it is a sign that you are working out too hard and need to slow your pace or exercise for less time. It does not mean that you should not exercise.

Back Pain

We have not included the story of any of our many patients with back pain. You probably can substitute your own story, because 80 percent of us have or will have back pain sometime in our lives. As you are reading this section, it is even more likely that you already are in that 80 percent. Luckily, most back pain gets better on its own. Once your back stops hurting, it is time to start exercising to keep the pain from coming back.

Back Anatomy 101 (for Nonscience Majors)

The spinal column is an amazing structure. It is sturdy enough to keep you upright, flexible enough for you to touch your toes (for some of you, that is), and built to protect the spinal cord's delicate nerve fibers. Your spine is divided into three major regions: the cervical (neck), thoracic (chest), and lumbar (low back) spine (see Figure 4.4).

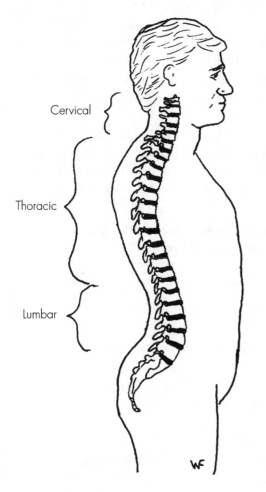

Cervical

Thoracic

Lumbar

WF

Figure 4.4   The three major anatomic regions of the spine.

The cervical spine consists of the top seven vertebrae of your neck. These bones are numbered, from the head down, as C-1 through C-7. The neck bones are smaller and move more freely, allowing your head to turn. Next are the 12 vertebrae of the thoracic spine. They connect to your ribs, which encircle your lungs and hold the thoracic spine in place. The supporting rib cage is why backaches are rare in the thoracic spine. The next five vertebrae make up your lumbar spine. So called from the Latin root *lumbaranos,* which we think means waiting to inflict pain when least expected. (Please note that the backbone is connected to the pelvic bone, not the hip bone.)

What's Hurting?

All along its length, the spinal column has four components: (1) vertebrae (your back bones), (2) facet joints between your back bones, (3) disks between the vertebral bodies, and (4) supporting muscles and ligaments. Eighty percent of back pain is due to problems with the muscles, disks, and facet joints. Although most back pain is self-limited, certain symptoms (listed in Table 4.8) should have you calling your health care provider.

Your back bones, or vertebrae, surround the spinal cord. The thick cylindrical body of a vertebra can become compressed (like stepping on an empty soda can) when your bones are thinned by osteoporosis. It is this compression and loss in height that results in the bent-forward

---

TABLE 4.8 **When to Seek Immediate Care for Your Back Pain**

See your health care provider if you have back pain plus any of the following:

- Unexplained weight loss or a past history of cancer
- Recent trauma to your back
- Weakness in your leg(s) or trouble urinating or moving your bowels
- Use of cortisone or corticosteroids
- Fever of more than 100°F or a condition increasing your risk of infection (such as a urinary catheter or having suppressed immunity)
- Intravenous drug use
- Symptoms lasting longer than four weeks
- Need to document the extent of an injury, as when litigation may be involved

posture of many elderly women. To allow movement, each vertebra is connected by two facet joints to the vertebra above and by two more joints to the vertebra below. As you twist and bend, each of your top 24 vertebrae interlock, for a total of 46 joints. Just like any other joint, these tiny facet joints can be sprained or strained.

The vertebral bodies are separated by disks, which act as shock absorbers for your spine. The disks have a tough fibrous coating and a softer interior, a little like a jelly donut. After about age 20, your disks start becoming stale—they become drier and stiffer. Then, if the disk suddenly is stressed, its jelly-like interior can push out the side in what is called a disk herniation. (Disks do not "slip" out of place, but their contents can get displaced.) The blown out portion of the disk can press on your nerves where they enter or leave your spinal canal. Depending on which disk is involved, the nearby nerves may be headed to your arm (if the cervical spine is affected) or your leg (if the disk is in your lumbar spine). Pressure on the nerve causes pain down your arm or leg, even though the problem is in your back.

Your muscles and ligaments are the fourth part of the spine. Muscles run lengthwise in front of and behind your back bones. Located behind your spine, the *extensor* muscles straighten your back. In front, the *flexors* bend your spine forward. Unlike your limbs, which have joint movement controlled by a few large muscles, the spine is supported by many smaller muscles, each spanning only one or two vertebral bodies. Like a stadium wave, these muscles must be coordinated precisely for smooth, painless spinal movement. If one of your back muscles is injured, it can go into spasm, which disrupts the coordination needed for back motion. Any attempt at movement only adds to the muscle imbalance and makes the back pain worse.

Piriformis syndrome is a common cause for "pain in the butt." The piriformis muscle is deep in your buttock. If the muscle is over worked, it can go into spasm. This causes pain in the center of your buttock, and because the muscle pinches your sciatic nerve, pain can shoot down the back of your leg. Icing the muscle and specific stretches will help relax the muscle and remedy the problem.

A Workout a Day Helps Keep Your Backache Away

Immediately after a back injury, you may feel that all you can do is lie in bed with an ice pack wedged under your spine. Do not stay there too long. Studies show that your back pain improves just as fast when you are up and moving around. By staying active, as best you can, the rest of your body will not become deconditioned.

Once you are pain free, you can begin a regular exercise routine to strengthen the spine's supporting muscles. Both strengthening your

You can apply cold to your back by filling a Dixie cup with water and putting it in the freezer. When the water is frozen, peel back the top edge, and you have an ice massager. A wet towel, frozen woody hard, also works well to ice your back.

Exercises to strengthen your back and abdominal muscles will create a muscular corset to protect your spine.

Golf and racquet sports are notorious for causing back pain. To avoid backaches, it is important to get coaching on the correct form and to warm up well and stretch before you tee off or start a match.

back muscles and increasing your overall endurance can help keep your backache from coming back. Back exercises have been used for years, but there is surprisingly little scientific evidence to know how well they work. Both exercises that flex (Williams exercises) and extend (MacKenzie exercises) your spine have their advocates. Specific exercises are illustrated in Figure 4.5. We recommend a progression of both flexion and extension exercises, focusing on those that provide the best pain relief.

In addition to back exercises, regular aerobic or endurance training can help prevent back problems. In fact, improving your fitness may be more important than using back exercises. The general advice on starting an exercise program in Chapter 12 applies to you if you have a history of back pain. What is different, though, is that some aerobic exercises may be better than others. Check Table 4.9 to compare different types of aerobic training.

If Your Back Pain Does Not Go Away

Almost 90 percent of back pain is better in one month. For a few unfortunate people, back pain becomes chronic and lasts more than six weeks. By that time, an additional set of problems has been added. The back pain can have unhealthy effects on your body mechanics. In addition, you are probably worried about your ability to work and about medical expenses. Also, a person with chronic back pain may have unknowingly become drug dependent from trying to mask the pain without correcting the underlying cause. Too often, a back operation is considered to be the next step. Surgery may be the right thing to do, or it may be time to see a *back team.* Often, the team is lead by a physiatrist (a physician specializing in musculoskeletal disorders and rehabilitation), and other team members may be physical and occupational therapists, orthopedic physicians or neurosurgeons, pain specialists, social workers, and psychologists.

Final Comments

For most individuals with arthritis, exercise can be an important component of their care. A joint that is acutely injured needs rest (along

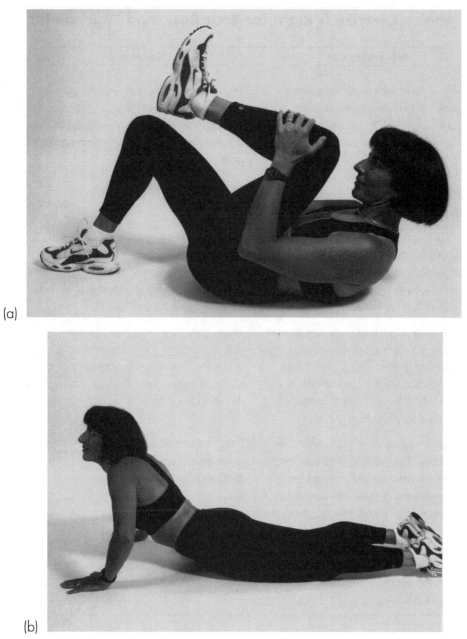

(a)

(b)

Figure 4.5   Examples of flexion (a, Williams) and extension (b, MacKenzie) back exercises.

TABLE 4.9   **Which Exercise Is Right for Your Back and Your Joints?**

Exercise	Advantages	Cautions
Swimming	Strengthens the upper body, and water's buoyancy prevents jarring or bouncing of your joints and spine. Using the hot tub after a swim can reduce muscle pain. The Arthritis Foundation sponsors water aerobics classes. Floatation belts and vests can further reduce joint stress when getting started or when leg joints are painful.	The crawl and breaststroke can force the back to arch, which may cause back pain for some people. Use a mask and snorkel to breathe if you have cervical spine arthritis or pain.
Biking	Improves muscular endurance, especially in the legs. When choosing a bike, have an expert help you select a bike that fits correctly.	When not on a stationary cycle, wear a helmet. Off-roading on a mountain bike risks the trauma of a fall on a rough road or trail.
Walking and running	Walking is the most popular exercise. Using your arms (power walking) with an exaggerated swing or carrying hand-held weights can increase the intensity of your workout, without increasing your pace.	Jogging on concrete sidewalks wearing shoes with poor support will jackhammer your back and joints. Invest in a top-quality pair of cushioned shoes and use level trails, grass, or a padded track.
Weight lifting or strength training	Depending on the weights lifted, the number of repetitions, and how long you rest between sets, weight lifting can cause a greater improvement in either muscular endurance or strength. Machines usually are safer than free weights. Get instruction and initial coaching from a physical therapist or certified trainer. Warm up and stretch before a workout.	Lifting with improper technique or lifting too much weight can cause back and joint problems

with ice, elevation, and a compression bandage [see page 267). For chronic degenerative arthritis, the prescription is exercise. Maintaining the strength of tissues surrounding the joint will decrease its further damage. For some, bracing or specific advice to remedy mechanical problems can also help protect already-damaged joints. Regular physical activity is important for those with inflammatory arthritis, too. Often a physical medicine doctor or knowledgeable physical therapist can help tailor exercises for your particular needs. Because parts of your body other than your joints can be affected by inflammatory arthritis, it is best to check with your health care provider before beginning your training program.

Most of us have or will have back pain. Nevertheless, your back is a sturdy structure and resilient to most injuries. You do not need to wait for a problem to use regular physical activity to avoid a backache. Maintaining your fitness through regular aerobic exercise and strengthening the muscles supporting your back are the best ways to prevent back problems.

Chapter 5

Exercise to Prevent and Treat Diabetes

Around 600 B.C., just a few years before we finished medical school, Indian physicians observed that the sugar content of their diabetic patients' urine was reduced with exercise. (You can only imagine how they checked for urine sweetness 2,600 years ago.) Not to be outdone by these earlier observations, in 1997 the American Diabetes Association recommended that people with diabetes include "exercise . . . for 20–45 minutes at least 3 days a week." The American College of Sports Medicine advises more exercise for those with diabetes and encourages 30 minutes or more of moderate physical activity each day of the week. We side with the sports medicine group for several reasons. Since exercise can improve blood sugar among those with diabetes, why use the treatment only three days per week? Come on now! Doctors do not prescribe most medications to be taken only three times per week. Three days of exercise each week is fine to improve low levels of fitness, but not sufficient to treat a disorder of your body's metabolism. The second reason is that we know doctors. Rarely have we seen a diabetes expert in top physical shape. Go to a Diabetes Association meeting and look for yourself. Then travel to an American College of Sports Medicine meeting. You will be surprised. You won't find many people at the sports medicine meeting because they are all out exercising—running through the streets, walking around the city, or lifting weights in the hotel fitness center.

There are approximately 16 million Americans with diabetes. Another 10 million have abnormal sugar metabolism (called glucose intolerance or borderline diabetes), which increases the risk of developing full-blown diabetes.

Slowly but surely his weight had been creeping upward—four pounds one year, three pounds the next. Mike Daniels, a 48-year-old salesman, who says he can "sell anything to anyone," was the heaviest he had ever been. Over the past 10 years, he gained a grand total of 37 pounds. What was once a 5 foot 10 inch, 160 pound man with a 33 inch waist, turned into a 197 pound man with a 39 inch waist. He went from the middleweight boxing division to a weight greater than many heavyweight champions, including Jack Dempsey and Rocky Marciano.

Mike has a six-year history of high blood pressure, treated with three medications. His sons (all five of them) were athletes, and he enjoyed watching them participate in sports. But he always claimed, "I'm just too busy to exercise." At the doctor's office for his annual exam, he complained of being thirsty much of the time, and drinking so much water that he woke 5 to 10 times each night. During the day he was also a frequent visitor to the bathroom—and he kept drinking fluids because he remained so thirsty. In addition, he complained that his toes felt "a little numb and tingling," and his vision seemed to become blurred at times.

He wondered if this was just middle age catching up with him. After his examination and blood tests, he was informed that he had Type 2 diabetes (formerly called adult-onset diabetes): his blood sugar (glucose) level was 308 mg/dL (normal is 60 to 110 mg/dL).

Americans have a one in nine chance of developing diabetes. Diabetes claims 178,000 lives each year and is the leading cause of blindness.

Fifty-six years old and an avid exerciser, Libby has competed in many road races and several marathons. She has required insulin to control her blood sugar for the past 22 years, since testing revealed she had Type 1 (insulin-dependent, previously known as juvenile-onset) diabetes mellitus. She remains meticulous about monitoring her blood sugar because she knows that her body needs a lower dose when she exercises. If she did not decrease the insulin injection, her blood sugar would drop, possibly to a dangerously low level.

When exercising, Libby brings along graham crackers and juice, stored in a fanny pack, to give her a sugar boost before it becomes dangerously low. Over the past few weeks Libby has been concerned about chest discomfort, especially at night while lying in bed and watching television. She described it as a dull pain, often associated with belching and an acid taste in the back of her throat. At the same time, Libby has been having new problems with blood sugar control. Her glucose sometimes drops to very low levels (below 60 mg/dL) and does not respond as quickly as before to a simple carbohydrate snack. When she cuts back on insulin, sometimes her blood sugar level climbs to the 300 mg/dL range or more.

Diabetes costs the people of the United States $92 billion each year.

What Is Diabetes?

Home sweet home, sugar, and *sweetie,* are all terms of endearment but a high blood sugar level is not. Diabetes mellitus is a disorder of sugar (also known as glucose) metabolism—our blood is too sweet for our own good. Diabetes is diagnosed by finding a high blood glucose level. Failure to regulate blood sugar is due either to a lack of insulin or to our body's insufficient response to the insulin we produce. These two distinct problems make up the two major categories of diabetes. Those with Type 1 diabetes (like Libby) require injections of insulin. Most people with Type 2 diabetes (like Mike), do not need insulin injections, but may require oral medications to help control their blood sugar levels.

Insulin is a hormone produced in the pancreas that guides sugar into cells and helps convert it into energy.

There is another category of abnormal sugar metabolism. *Stress diabetes* is diagnosed when a high blood sugar level is associated with a certain condition, such as pregnancy, diseases of the adrenal gland or pancreas, or use of medications, especially cortisone and water pills (diuretics). This form of diabetes often disappears when the stress is relieved.

Symptoms of Diabetes

The typical symptoms that can alert you and your doctor to the diagnosis of diabetes are known as the three polys (*poly* means many or a lot): polyphagia (eating), polydypsia (drinking), and polyuria (urination). When glucose levels in the blood climb over 180 mg/dL, the excess sugar begins to be dumped into the urine, causing the need for more water to be eliminated. This excess urine production can make you dehydrated and leads to dizziness and excessive thirst and hunger (polydypsia and polyphagia). These classic symptoms and other potential indications that you may have diabetes are listed in Table 5.1.

High blood sugar levels cause swelling of the lens of the eye, resulting in blurred vision. Nerves become swollen, producing numbness and/or a tingling sensation in the feet and hands. Because Type 2 diabetes evolves slowly, many people have no symptoms despite high blood sugar levels.

TABLE 5.1   **First Symptoms of Diabetes**

Symptoms	Type 1 Diabetes	Type 2 Diabetes
Increased hunger	Yes	Yes
Increased thirst	Yes	Yes
Increased urination	Yes	Yes
Weight loss	Yes	Yes
Lightheaded feeling	Yes	Yes
Bladder and vaginal infections	No	Yes
Numbness and/or tingling of hands and feet	Less common	Yes
Blurred vision	Less common	Yes
No symptoms	No	Yes

Diagnosing Diabetes

There are several ways to diagnose diabetes. One is an oral glucose toler-ance test. This test requires you to drink 75 grams of a very thick, sugary solution over a maximum of five minutes. This is like having 15 tea-spoons of maple syrup—but without the waffles. After swallowing, blood sugar levels are tested over the next few hours. If the plasma glucose is 190 mg/dL one hour after drinking the solution, or more than 140 mg/dL, two hours after drinking the ultrasweet concoction, the diagnosis of dia-betes is made. Once a common procedure, the glucose tolerance test is now used mainly to determine pregnancy-associated diabetes. Usually, the results do not add much to your fasting blood sugar levels. To be ac-curate, people need to be "primed" by eating and drinking sugary foods and liquids for several days prior to the test, otherwise the results may be unreliable and falsely label you as having diabetes.

In the United States there are 800,000 people diagnosed with diabetes each year.

Today, diabetes is usually determined by checking your blood sugar level after an eight-hour fast or two hours after a meal. If the level is 200 mg/dL after eating, or above 126 mg/dL (fasting) for two separate tests, it is highly likely that you have diabetes.

The glycosylated hemoglobin (or hemoglobin A_1C) test can strengthen the diagnosis. Hemoglobin A_1C values represent the aver-age blood sugar levels over the past 8 to 12 weeks. If the value is ele-vated, the diagnosis of diabetes is usually confirmed. Table 5.2 lists methods of diagnosing diabetes.

TABLE 5.2 **Diabetes Diagnosis**	
Diagnosis	**Glucose Levels (mg/dL)**
Normal	Below 110 (fasting)
Impaired control (borderline)	110–125 (fasting)
Probable diabetes	126 +
Diabetes	Symptoms (the three P's) and
	200+ (nonfasting)
	or
	126+ (fasting) twice
	or
	200+ (two hours after a meal)

Causes of Type 1 and Type 2 Diabetes

Type 1 diabetes most often occurs among children and young adults and is usually due to an overactivity of the body's immune system that results in the destruction of insulin-producing cells within the pancreas, leading to a total deficiency of insulin. With no insulin, there is no control of blood sugar. With Type 1 diabetes, insulin injections are required, not only to control symptoms (Table 5.1), but to keep you alive.

When is an apple not healthy? When you are shaped like one. Upper body fat causes your insulin to be less effective and increases your risk for heart disease.

Type 2 diabetes, formerly referred to as adult-onset diabetes, is nearly 20 times more common than Type 1. There are a number of factors (Table 5.3) that increase your risk of developing this form of diabetes. This type of diabetes is often related to our lifestyles. Those with Type 2 diabetes still produce their own insulin. In fact, insulin levels can be higher than normal. The problem is that the insulin produced is not very effective because of the body's resistance to insulin's sugar-lowering effects.

Type 2 diabetes makes up nearly 95 percent of all cases of diabetes mellitus. Nearly 90 percent of people with Type 2 diabetes are overweight.

Instead of insulin injections, those with Type 2 diabetes can often control their symptoms and blood sugar levels by diet, exercise, and medications that improve the function of insulin. Overall, the risk of developing Type 2 diabetes increases with age, higher body weight (over 120 percent of ideal), lack of exercise, a diet rich in high-fat foods, and a family history of diabetes.

TABLE 5.3   **Factors That Increase Your
Risk of Developing Diabetes**

Not exercising
Eating too much fat
Being overweight (20 pounds or more)
Family history of diabetes
Getting older

What Controls Your Blood Sugar?

Insulin is the main hormone that controls the entry of sugar from the bloodstream into the cells of our body. This hormone is produced by specialized beta cells, clustered in an area known as the islets of Langerhans in the pancreas. (After first hearing about these islets in medical school, we thought about vacationing there. But space is a problem, it's dark, and miniaturization has not yet been perfected.) Your body's insulin output from the pancreas is stimulated as blood sugar rises. Sugar levels increase when you eat food or drink calorie-containing liquids, especially when they contain carbohydrates (sugars and starches). Glucose levels also increase when you break down the stored carbohydrate in your liver.

In a person without diabetes, insulin production is balanced with the liver's breakdown of glycogen and production of new sugar, which usually keeps the body's blood glucose levels constant (usually between 60 and 110 mg/dL).

You function best when there is a normal level of blood sugar. If your levels are too high (a condition known as hyperglycemia), it signals that your cells are starving for energy, because the glucose swimming in your bloodstream is not able to be used. If your blood sugar level is too low (a condition known as hypoglycemia), there may not be enough glucose to allow your brain to function normally. When you don't eat, your liver, which stores carbohydrates (as glycogen), breaks them down to supply the rest of your body with glucose.

Problems Resulting from Diabetes

Over time, the body reacts to diabetes with an increased risk of cardiovascular problems (heart attacks, strokes), kidney failure, disease of the eye (retina), higher blood pressure, and elevated blood cholesterol and triglyceride levels. The longer a person has diabetes, the greater risk of developing these problems. Table 5.4 lists some of the common long-term complications of diabetes.

What Do Carbohydrate Foods Do for People with Diabetes?

There are basically two kinds of carbohydrates: simple and complex. All carbohydrates are sugar molecules. When only one or two sugar molecules are linked together, as in table sugar (sucrose), milk (lactose), or typical sport drinks and soda pop (fructose), we have simple carbohydrates. When you eat or drink simple carbohydrates, they are quickly absorbed from your gastrointestinal tract and enter the bloodstream, supplying your body with immediate energy. Because of this swift absorption, insulin levels must increase rapidly. If the insulin level does not immediately increase, as in those with diabetes, the blood sugar level soars upward. Eating simple carbohydrates can help someone with diabetes who has hypoglycemia (a low blood sugar level) due

---

TABLE 5.4 **Effects of Diabetes on the Body**

Body Part	Complication
Eye (retina)	May result in blindness
Kidney	May result in protein loss and kidney failure
Nerves	Gastrointestinal tract (bloating, nausea, diarrhea, heartburn), blood pressure problems (dizziness with standing), and numbness and tingling or burning pain of the hands and feet
Muscles	Weakness and loss of muscle mass
Blood vessels	More rapid development of arteriosclerosis resulting in narrowed blood vessels and reduced blood supply to the brain and extremities. People with diabetes who are 60 years of age and older have up to five times the risk of suffering a stroke. Restricted blood flow can result in ulcers of the feet, which may lead to infection and amputation.
Cardiac	Heart attacks and reduced blood flow to the heart

to the use of too much insulin, excess oral medication, or long and strenuous exercise. Simple carbohydrates can almost immediately boost blood sugar levels to a safe range.

When several sugar molecules are linked together in chains, as in rice, breads, and cereals, they are referred to as complex carbohydrates. These carbohydrates are absorbed more slowly and provide energy over a longer period of time. Eating complex carbohydrates will not cause as great a surge in the body's production of insulin, and is less likely to cause rapid increases in blood sugar among those with diabetes. Thus, complex carbohydrates are the preferred dietary form of sugar.

Exercise and Carbohydrates

Carbohydrates are the body's high-octane fuel and the only energy source that can be used during intense exercise. Once in your blood-stream, sugar is used by your cells for energy or is stored as the substance glycogen in your muscles and liver. Glycogen is your body's fuel tank for high-octane sugar. However, there is a difference between the liver and muscle storage tanks. The glycogen stored in your liver can be broken down to glucose and provide energy for the rest of your body. The glycogen in your muscle is locked into that particular muscle and can be used only by that muscle group for exercise. It cannot break down and reenter your bloodstream to be used by other cells.

A Diet You Can Live With

Food choices are vital to controlling blood sugar. The food you eat affects both the dose of insulin and the potential complications of diabetes. Although the old phrase, "you are what you eat," is not necessarily true in all cases, "you become what you eat" is more fitting, especially for those with diabetes. Your food selections can help you delay or even prevent the disabling effects of diabetes, such as kidney disease, high blood pressure, abnormal cholesterol and triglyceride levels, slow stomach emptying (a condition known as gastroparesis), and heart disease.

If you have diabetes you have many food choices—there is no one best diet for diabetes. Diets with exchange lists are available through the American Diabetes Association, registered dietitians, your physician's office, and local hospitals. However, the basics of a so-called diabetic diet are the basics of a healthy diet for everyone: eat less fat and simple carbohydrate (sugary) foods, consume fresh fruits and vegetables, and eat only lean meats such as chicken, turkey, and fish. A general diet plan is listed in Table 5.5.

Eat at consistent times each day so that you match your food intake to when your insulin and/or oral medications are most effective (Table 5.5). Then check your glucose levels to find how you might change the insulin or oral medication dose to match the quantity and type of foods you are eating.

> The yearly health costs for people with diabetes are nearly four times those of people without diabetes.

Using Insulin

Type 1 diabetes requires injectable insulin therapy. There are approximately 30 different types of insulin. Although all types lower blood sugar, they have different speeds of onset, time to peak glucose lowering, and duration of activity (how long the effect lasts). Several examples of insulin that you may be using are listed in Table 5.6.

Some regular insulin is mixed in the same bottle with NPH insulin in a specified proportion, to avoid the need to take two separate injections. The mix is often 70/30, that is, 70 percent NPH insulin and 30 percent regular insulin. It is not wise to combine regular with Lente insulin because the mixture will cause regular insulin to turn into Lente, with a longer duration of activity. Exercise increases the speed of onset and the blood-sugar-lowering effect of all types of insulin.

> There are an estimated 500,000 to 1 million people with Type 1 diabetes in the United States.

TABLE 5.5 **Recommended Diets for Diabetes**

1. Total daily calories from fat should be 30 percent or less.
2. If overweight, reduce the fat calories to 20 percent.
3. Total daily calories from carbohydrates should be 50 to 60 percent.
4. Carbohydrates should be mainly fruits and starches (breads, rice, pasta), not candies, fruit juice, or soda pop.
5. Eat a variety of vegetables for their vitamins, minerals, and fiber.
6. Don't fry your food; bake, broil, steam, or poach instead.
7. Eat most calories during the time of peak insulin or other diabetes medication action.

	(time in hours)		
Insulin	Time to Onset	Greatest Effect	Duration Effect
Lispro	1/4–1/2	1/2–1 1/2	3–5
Regular	1/2–1	2–3	6–8
NPH	1–2	5–8	18–28
Lente	1–3	6–8	18–28
Ultralente	3–4	9–15	22–30

TABLE 5.6 **Action of Types of Insulin**

What Does Exercise Do to Sugar and the Action of Insulin?

Any change in the effect of insulin action will affect blood sugar. About 75 years ago, an experiment showed how physical activity boosts the effect of insulin. A patient was given a dose of 10 units of regular insulin, and his blood sugar level was followed as it gradually lowered over the next several hours. On another day, the subject was given the same dose of insulin and began to exercise. The effect was dramatic. With the addition of exercise, the level of sugar dropped like a rock! Exercise literally supercharged the injected insulin.

There are two major reasons this occurred. First, insulin is absorbed from the injection site more rapidly during exercise, so its sugar-lowering effects occur faster. Secondly, an exercising muscle acts like a high-powered vacuum cleaner, sucking up sugar molecules to use as fuel, even if just a small amount of insulin is around.

Although this 1926 experiment was the first to show how exercise can assist insulin in the treatment of diabetes, here is a note of caution: it is important that people who exercise and use insulin plan their activities and insulin dose based on (1) when the exercise will occur (exercising at peak insulin effect is more likely to cause very low blood sugar levels), (2) how long the exercise will be (the longer the exercise, the greater the blood-sugar-lowering effect), (3) how intense the exercise will be (the harder the exertion, the lower the blood sugar level), and (4) how much carbohydrate snack to carry (to avoid an excessively low blood sugar level [hypoglycemia]). Even with the best planning, hypoglycemia can occur. So, always carry carbohydrate snacks to avoid and treat it.

Besides the immediate effects of exercise on insulin, those who have Type 2 diabetes and exercise regularly have better overall control of their blood sugar levels. This is due to the improvement in the body's sensitivity to insulin. With regular exercise, the uptake of glucose and breakdown of glycogen are increased. Also, physical training among people with diabetes improves cholesterol and triglyceride levels. Since those with diabetes are at much higher risk for heart and blood vessel disease, this effect is extremely important.

Hypoglycemia is a medical emergency. A very low blood sugar level requires immediate treatment. If you have diabetes, always carry 10 to 20 grams of simple carbohydrate (4 ounces of juice, candy, or sugar tablets).

Will Exercise Reduce My Risk of Developing Diabetes?

Although exercise does not prevent Type 1 diabetes, it can aid treatment. In fact, before insulin's discovery in the earlier part of this century, physical activity was a cornerstone of diabetes therapy. On the other hand, you are much less likely to develop Type 2 diabetes when you exercise regularly. This benefit was shown by researchers in Sweden, who followed people with mild or borderline Type 2 diabetes for six years. Half of the group received advice about their diet and began a walking program. They exercised for a total of two hours each week. The others did not exercise. At the conclusion of the study, only half as many of the exercisers had evidence of diabetes.

How does exercise prevent diabetes? Good question! There seems to be several ways this occurs. Even after as little as six weeks of regular physical activity there are signs that insulin is more effective. Your body becomes more sensitive to insulin's action, so that sugar is more easily removed from the bloodstream and blood glucose levels can normalize. Also, regular exercise can help you prevent the typical one to two pound weight gain that occurs each year after age 21. By limiting weight gains and improving the effectiveness of your own insulin, you reduce your risk of developing Type 2 diabetes.

People between the ages of 40 and 84 who report exercising vigorously at least once each week are leaner and have less Type 2 diabetes after five years.

The bottom line is that people who are better conditioned do not require their body's beta cells in the pancreas to produce as much insulin. However, those who are inactive make demands on their pancreas to pump out the insulin. This not only increases cardiovascular risk factors, it may fatigue our beta cells. This may be one reason why older, sedentary people are more likely to develop Type 2 diabetes. Their insulin-producing beta cells are just wearing out.

Treating Type 2 Diabetes

Type 2 diabetes is treated with exercise, diet, often with oral medication, and sometimes with insulin. There are several types of oral drugs (Table 5.7), and each category has its own unique features. Often these drugs are combined to improve control of blood sugar.

There are many reasons to use exercise in the treatment of diabetes. As you may remember from the earlier portion of the chapter (unless you skipped ahead to start reading, as we often do), the effect of insulin is improved with each workout. This is due to increased absorption of insulin from the injection site and greater uptake of blood sugar into your working muscles. After 1½ to 4 months of regular exercise your body becomes more sensitive to the sugar-lowering effect of insulin, even at rest. This makes it possible to treat diabetes (Type 1) with less insulin or reduce the output of insulin from the pancreas

Of all the therapies suggested for diabetes management (insulin, sulfonylureas, biguanide therapy, acarbose, and exercise), only acarbose and exercise are not associated with weight gain.

TABLE 5.7 Oral Drugs Used to Treat Type 2 Diabetes

Drug Class	Examples	Action
Sulfonylureas	Tolbutamide (Orinase), glipizide (Glucotrol), glyburide (Micronase, Diabeta, Glynase), glimepiride (Amaryl)	Increases insulin output from the pancreas
Biguanide	Metformin (Glucophage)	Lowers sugar production in the liver; increases insulin activity
Alpha glucosidase inhibitor	Acarbose (Precose)	Delays sugar absorption from the intestines; increases insulin activity
Thiazolidinediones	Troglitazone (Rezulin), Rosiglitazone (Avandia), Proglitazone (Actos)	Increases insulin activity
Meglitinides	Repaglinide (Prandin)	Increases insulin output from the pancreas

(Type 2 diabetes), because of the supercharging effect of exercise on insulin. This is very important, since the lowering of insulin levels reduces the risk for heart disease, high blood pressure, and obesity.

Exercise to Prevent Diabetes

The most common and most preventable form of diabetes is that which comes with being overweight and inactive. Blood tests on sedentary and obese people often show elevated blood sugar levels during stressful situations. The reason this occurs is that they are becoming resistant to the effects of insulin. The blood sugar level may be normal without the stress, but only because the pancreas is pumping out high amounts of insulin. When the stress calls for even more insulin, the pancreas just cannot produce.

Type 2 diabetes can be prevented by regular exercise, especially when a person's diet remains healthy. But as with all prevention, you need to start early. You don't get a chance to prevent diabetes after you develop it. And 800,000 new cases of diabetes each year attest to the problem. You can help lower this statistic. If you want to find out if you are at high risk to develop Type 2 diabetes, look again at Table 5.3.

By exercising 30 minutes at least four times each week (Table 5.8) at moderate intensity (a heart rate of 70 to 85 percent of your maximal rate, or exercising to a level that allows you to talk but not to sing during the activity), you reduce your chances of developing blood sugar problems and increase the effectiveness of your body's insulin. This is adequate for prevention, but daily exercise is best for treatment of diabetes. The formula in Table 5.8 is useful for most people who want to find their appropriate exercise heart rate.

Exercise is like a medication. Although you can improve your physical capacity by exercising just three times a week for 20 minutes, you gain extra health benefits and extra calorie burning with more exercise. Most studies that fail to show health benefits of exercise are likely to include inadequate amounts of training. A prominent diabetes prevention study shows that two hours of weekly exercise reduces the risk of developing Type 2 diabetes by 50 percent! That means nearly 400,000 people each year could avoid developing Type 2 diabetes.

TABLE 5.8 **Exercise to Prevent and Treat Type 2 Diabetes**

How hard should I train?

1. Find your *maximal* heart rate:

     My maximal exercise heart rate = 220 − my age

     Enter your maximal heart rate:_____ beats/minute

2. Find your *training* heart rate:

     My training heart rate range = .7 to .85 × my maximal heart rate

     Enter your training heart rate: _____ to _____ beats/minute

Or choose the Borg Perceived Exertion Scale

Borg Perceived Exertion Scale

Number Rating	How the Exercise Feels to You
0	Nothing
0.5	Very, very weak
1	Very weak
2	Weak
3	Moderate
4	Somewhat strong
5	Strong
6	
7	Very strong
8	
9	
10	Maximal (can't do more)

Select exercise level 2 to 4

     How long and how many days each week should I exercise?

     A minimum of 30 minutes, four times each week

Do I Need to Visit My Health Care Provider before I Start to Exercise?

If you have diabetes, yes, you must see your health care provider before you start exercising. This is critical if the exercise is more than casual walking. Because people who have had diabetes for more than five years have a higher likelihood of cardiovascular disease, it is important to have a thorough examination prior to initiating an exercise program.

The medical history and physical examination should pay special attention to your heart, blood vessels, kidneys, nervous system, and eyes. Your health practitioner should include the points listed in Table 5.9.

When to Seek Advice

Because diabetes can cause diseases that can increase the risks of exercise, such as heart rhythm irregularities, it is important to know when not to exercise or when to ask your health care provider for advice or an exam (Table 5.10). The amount of exercise you can safely perform can be learned after your examination. For example, vigorous exertion should be avoided if there is a specific eye problem called proliferative retinopathy. Until the condition is treated and stabilized, extreme caution is necessary because bleeding in the retina may occur, resulting in blindness. If there is what is termed *background retinopathy of the eye*, low-impact exercise including walking, slow jogging, and cycling at

---

TABLE 5.9   **Medical Screening before Exercise**

Diabetes evaluation:

1. Eye exam (to evaluate your retina)
2. Nervous system exam (to check for nerve damage)
3. Measure your body composition (to check percentage of body fat)
4. Examine extremities, especially the feet
5. Urinalysis (to check for protein and sugar)
6. Kidney function tests (blood urea nitrogen and creatinine)
7. Blood glucose and glycated hemoglobin (hemoglobin A_{1c}) levels

Cardiovascular evaluation:

1. Blood pressure check, seated and standing
2. Evaluation of pulses (neck, groin, and feet)
3. Cholesterol and triglyceride levels
4. Electrocardiogram (EKG)
5. Exercise test if heart disease is present, you are over age 40, or have two or more cardiac risk factors (risk factors include abnormal cholesterol levels, high blood pressure, cigarette smoking, history of early heart disease in a close relative, and diabetes)

TABLE 5.10   **When to Seek Advice**

Don't exercise, instead see your doctor if you say yes to one of the following:

Do you have chest discomfort with exertion or at rest?
Do you have trouble breathing when you exercise?
Do you become dizzy when you exercise?
Do you have pains in your legs when you walk?
Is your blood sugar out of control?
Do you have sores on your feet that are not healing?
Has your vision suddenly worsened?

---

lower exercise zones (around 70 percent of maximal heart rate) is recommended. This level of exertion will not raise blood pressure very much and will therefore reduce the chance of eye damage.

Monitoring Your Sugar: Is Your Blood Too Sweet or Not Sweet Enough to Exercise?

You should always monitor your blood sugar level whether you are exercising or not. However, it is vital that you monitor your blood sugar level just before exercise, during physical activity (at 30 minute intervals), and at least 15 minutes after training. Check your urine for ketones (present when sugar control is very poor) if it has been difficult to regulate your blood sugar, because this will reveal an inadequate effect of insulin.

Don't begin exercise if your blood glucose level is (1) over 250 mg/dL (too sweet), (2) below 100 mg/dL (not sweet enough), or (3) if ketones are present in your urine. If your blood sugar is too high before exercise, your control is poor and your muscles are probably more resistant to using the circulating glucose. At the same time, your liver continues to go merrily about its normal business of breaking down glycogen and producing even more blood sugar during the exercise, thinking that all this fuel is going to be used for muscle energy. Unfortunately, what happens is that your blood sugar level soars skyward.

Fats are fuels for low-intensity exercise, whereas carbohydrates are fuels for high-intensity exertion.

On the other hand, if your blood sugar level is low, there may be too much insulin effect, so that not enough sugar is available for exercise. Because physical activity supercharges your insulin, training under these conditions can result in a wide range of problems, from mild symptoms of hypoglycemia (Table 5.11) to a severely lowered glucose level, with the possibility of fainting, coma, seizures, and brain damage So, if your blood sugar is below 100 mg/dL, you need to eat some carbohydrate foods or drink a carbohydrate drink first.

Hypoglycemia can occur even hours after you have stopped exercising. Continue to monitor your glucose levels for at least 8 hours after training. In some cases, low blood sugar can occur more than 24 hours after long and vigorous exercise.

Avoiding Foot Injury

Foot injury caused by poor circulation is common. Also, because diabetes can cause a loss of sensation in your feet, it is critical that you inspect your feet each day and choose shoes that fit properly and have enough cushion. One of the most important ways to avoid irritation is to lubricate and protect the skin of your toes. Watch for blisters or sores that do not heal. These can result in infection or be the result of reduced blood flow. Always keep your feet clean. Fungus tends to grow where it is warm, wet, and dark. Avoid walking barefoot, especially out of doors where you are more apt to step on a sharp object, break your skin, and develop skin infections. Small infections may not be noticed because of numbness. Those that go untreated can lead to hospitalization and even loss of a limb.

TABLE 5.11	**Some Warning Symptoms of Low Blood Sugar Level**
	Sweating (feeling cold and clammy)
	Feeling shaky and nervous
	Feeling weak and faint
	Heart pounding
	Excessive hunger
	Headache

Exercise Treatment

How Much Exercise Do I Need to Treat Type 1 Diabetes?

For those with Type 1 diabetes, exercise does not always result in as many benefits as it does for those with Type 2 diabetes. Exercising fewer than three days each week is ineffective management. However, training three or more times each week improves fitness, and blood sugar levels are better regulated. In a study by Barbara Campaign and associates, children with Type 1 diabetes exercised for 25 minutes at 80 percent of their maximal heart rate, three times each week, for 12 weeks. Fasting blood sugar levels dropped 16 percent, and the marker for long-term sugar level control (hemoglobin A_1C) was reduced by an average of 10 percent. However, exercise at lower intensity may not have beneficial effects on blood sugar levels or improve the effectiveness of insulin.

For adults, regular exercise at about 70 percent of maximal heart rate or a level of 2 to 3 out of 10 on the perceived exertion scale can reduce fasting blood sugar and hemoglobin A_{1c} levels, although not all studies are in agreement. The differences in research findings may be due to differences in the design of the studies, or more likely, the type, intensity, and amount of time the research subjects spent exercising. Overall, there is an improvement in the effect of insulin after exercise, and this will reduce your insulin dose or increase the amount of food you can eat. In addition, other cardiovascular risk factors such as abnormal cholesterol and triglyceride levels can be lowered, and reducing even mild high blood pressure will further reduce the chance of developing other complications. Even small improvements can make a critical difference. For example, in a 1998 study of more than 1,500 people with diabetes, those with a blood pressure of 144/81 mmHg had significantly fewer cardiovascular problems than subjects with the slightly higher blood pressure of 148/85 mmHg.

The blood pressure goal for those with diabetes is no more than 135/85 mm Hg.

How Much Exercise Do I Need to Treat Type 2 Diabetes?

In contrast to the results from Type 1 diabetes research, regular exercise consistently improves blood sugar levels for those with Type 2 diabetes.

In fact, sugar uptake into muscle is improved by more than 30 to 35 percent with regular exercise, and this can make a big difference in control of your blood sugar. Although the liver's glycogen fuel tank is lowered for those with diabetes, this biological storage tank is re-expanded with regular physical activity. Also, muscle enzyme function is improved and causes even more muscle glycogen to be formed. Importantly, those who reduce their weight and body fat, while maintaining their exercise, show the best blood sugar control. The combination of diet and exercise works better for people with Type 2 diabetes when compared with either a diet or exercise alone.

If You Are Overweight

For those with Type 2 diabetes who are overweight, lower levels of exercise intensity are the best. This type of training burns fat and lowers triglyceride levels (a blood fat risk factor for cardiovascular disease that is often high among those with Type 2 diabetes). When your triglyceride level is lowered, you receive a double benefit as an increase in the heart-healthy and protective (HDL) cholesterol occurs. If you are in the overweight category, exert yourself at a level of 2 out of 10. This will enable you to build up your exercise capacity so you are able to exert yourself for 30 minutes, seven days each week (Table 5.12). For the most effective weight loss and improvement in your blood triglyceride and cholesterol levels, the amount of fat in your diet can be critical. Keep the fat content of your diet to 20 percent of total calories or less.

If You Are Not Overweight

For those with Type 2 diabetes who are not overweight, slightly higher intensity exercise, at 70 to 85 percent of maximal heart rate or level 3 to 4 of your perceived exertion, and/or participating in weight training

TABLE 5.12	**Treatment of Overweight Type 2 Diabetes**
Intensity:	60 to 70 percent maximal heart rate
	or
	Level 2 (Borg scale)
Duration:	30 or more minutes
Frequency:	4 to 7 days each week

TABLE 5.13	**Treatment of Normal-Weight Type 2 Diabetes**
Intensity:	70 to 85 percent maximal heart rate
	or
	Level 3 to 4 (Borg scale)
Duration:	30 or more minutes
Frequency:	4 to 7 days each week

can increase the effectiveness of insulin and improve your blood sugar control (Table 5.13). We suggest that you carve out some time to exercise every day of the week, for a minimum of 30 minutes. This will burn calories (close to a pound of fat's worth of calories each week) and better regulate your blood sugar. The end result will be reduced cardiovascular risk factors and a much lower risk of developing problems associated with diabetes.

Exercising at lower intensities, such as an intensity of 2 on the perceived exertion scale, can be effective for blood pressure control and keeping your weight down but is less likely to improve cholesterol levels if you are not overweight.

What about My Insulin Dose When I Exercise?

If diabetes is well controlled, it is important to decrease your insulin dose before you exercise because of the supercharging effect that physical activity has on insulin. Only your experience will help you discover the right amount of insulin to use. In general, lower your use of intermediate-acting (Lente or NPH) insulin by about 15 percent on days you exercise 30 or more minutes at low or moderate intensity. If you are using several doses of short-acting insulin (Table 5.14), reduce the pre-exercise amount, and monitor your blood sugar level after exercise. If you receive your insulin by a subcutaneous pump, eliminate the extra mealtime amount or the extra dose that comes before or after the physical activity. By using an exercise log, you will be able to determine the dosages necessary for you.

TABLE 5.14   **Dosage Changes of Regular Insulin Prior to Exercise (Guidelines for Those with Controlled Diabetes)**

Exercise Intensity*	Exercise Duration	Insulin Dose
Low	Less than 15 minutes	No change
Moderate	Less than 15 minutes	No change
Low	15 to 30 minutes	75 percent of regular
Moderate	15 to 30 minutes	50 percent of regular
Low	31 to 45 minutes	50 percent of regular
Moderate	31 to 45 minutes	25 percent of regular
Low	46 to 60 minutes	25 percent of regular
Moderate	46 to 60 minutes	No regular insulin

*Low intensity: training heart rate of 70 percent or less or a Borg scale of 0.5 to 2.

Moderate intensity: training heart rate of 70 to 80 percent or maximum or Borg scale of 3 to 4.

Table 5.14 provides a guide to help you estimate the changes needed in your regular (short-acting) insulin dose. Because each person's insulin dose and sensitivities are different, you will need to construct your own guide.

Table 5.15 is designed to help you use your pre-exercise blood sugar as a guide to adjusting your own insulin and diet, before and during exertion. Table 5.16 provides some examples of high-carbohydrate snacks.

Some Rules to Live By

In general, if your blood sugar is below 80 mg/dL, eat at least 15 grams of carbohydrate (3 graham crackers, 1/2 bagel, 1/2 banana, or 1 medium orange) (Table 5.16) prior to exercise and always wait until your blood sugar is above 100 mg/dL before exercising.

A few other rules to follow are (1) wear a medical bracelet that will inform people that you have diabetes (this is especially important if you have an insulin reaction and can't speak), (2) don't inject insulin into the limbs you will be exercising (this will increase the absorption of in-

TABLE 5.15 **Prevention of Hypoglycemia during Exercise (Examples)**

If Your Blood Sugar is	And Your Exercise Will Be	Eat	During Exercise Eat	Pre-exercise Snack Examples
Less than 100 mg/dL	Low to moderate intensity for 30 minutes or less	15 grams of carbohydrate	Often not necessary, may need another 15 grams immediately after exercise	1 fruit or bread exchange
Less than 100 mg/dL	Moderate intensity for more than 30 minutes	25 grams of carbohydrate	15 or more grams of carbohydrate each hour	$^1/_2$ sandwich with a fruit exchange or milk
Less than 100 mg/dL	High intensity	50 grams of carbohydrates	25 or more grams of carbohydrate each hour	1 sandwich with a fruit exchange
100 to 250 mg/dL	Low to moderate intensity, 30 minutes or less	Nothing before exercise	May not require any carbohydrate during exercise	
100 to 250 mg/dL	Moderate intensity for more than 30 minutes	Nothing before exercise	15 or more grams of carbohydrate each $^1/_2$ to 1 hour	
100 to 180 mg/dL	High intensity for 1 hour or more	25 to 50 grams of carbohydrates	15 or more grams of carbohydrate each $^1/_2$ hour to 1 hour	1 sandwich with a fruit or milk exchange
180 to 250 mg/dL	High intensity for 1 hour or more	Nothing before exercise	15 or more grams of carbohydrate each $^1/_2$ to 1 hour	

sulin and more rapidly lower blood sugar levels), (3) don't exercise at the time of peak insulin activity (see Table 5.6), and (4) guard against hypoglycemia. For vigorous training sessions that last one hour or more, check your blood sugar levels 15 minutes after exercise and every two hours for at least the next eight hours. If you have exercised long and hard, the carbohydrates you eat after exertion may be sucked right into the glycogen storage tanks in your muscle and liver. This can result in hypoglycemia, which can last for more than a day!

TABLE 5.16	**High-Carbohydrate Snacks for the Road (Examples)**
Item	**Carbohydrate Grams (Approximate)**
Apple (1 medium)	20
Grape juice (8 oz.)	25
Bagel (1)	30
Orange (1 medium)	15
Bread (1 slice)	15
Orange juice (8 oz.)	25
Cherries (10)	10
Pear	20
Fig bar (1)	10
Prunes (5 dried)	25
Graham crackers (1 square)	5
Raisins (seedless, 1/2 cup)	60
Grapes (1/2 cup)	20
Saltine crackers (5)	10
Sandwich (1)	30
Milk (8 oz.)	15

What about My Oral Diabetes Medication and Exercise?

If you are exercising more that 30 minutes at a moderate or high intensity, for example, at a Borg perceived exertion rating of 3 or more, you should reduce your oral medicine (if your sugar has been well controlled). Add extra carbohydrate before exercise if your blood sugar level is below 100 mg/dL. Since there are so many varieties of medication for Type 2 diabetes (Table 5.7), glucose monitoring is the best way to find out what works best for you.

Mike was determined not to be "licked" by diabetes. He wanted to know about his diet, whether he needed medicine, and how he could lower his chances of developing complications. He learned that the high sugar content of his blood caused more urine to be created and resulted in his frequent trips to the urinal. This left him dehydrated and thirsty much of the time. The visual blurriness was due to the swelling of the lens of his eye, because of poor glucose control, not due to potential problems with his retina.

His symptoms of numbness and tingling in his lower legs and the finding that he could not distinguish a sharp pin from a dull cotton swab touching the soles of his feet were symptoms of nerve impairment in his feet (called diabetic peripheral neuropathy). His cholesterol (320 mg/dL) and triglyceride (420 mg/dL) levels were high, which is common among newly diagnosed patients with Type 2 diabetes. His kidney function (blood urea nitrogen and creatinine) was normal, and his urinalysis was fine, without any protein present.

An exercise stress test with electrocardiogram monitoring was normal and Mike began a program of progressive walking along with taking one 81 mg coated aspirin each day. He closely inspected his feet before and after each daily walk. This was especially important because of his lower leg numbness. Within eight weeks Mike was walking three miles every day and had lost 10 pounds. His fasting blood sugar level, without medication, dropped to 140 mg/dL, and his triglyceride level decreased to 125 mg/dL. Because his cholesterol level remained elevated, he was treated with cholesterol-lowering medication.

Ten years later, Mike is walking five miles each day. He has maintained his 25 pound weight loss over the years. The tingling and numbness in his feet have subsided. Although he is still being treated for high blood pressure, it is well controlled with much less medication. He continues to manage his diabetes with diet and exercise and keeps on selling.

Mike Daniels may well have prevented or delayed the onset of his Type 2 diabetes with regular exercise. Since beginning his daily walks, modifying his diet, and losing weight, he has controlled his blood sugar levels, lowered his triglyceride levels and blood pressure, and achieved a fitter, healthier body. He continues to have normal yearly eye exams, and his kidney function has remained normal. Mike continues to take an 81 mg aspirin tablet each day to further reduce his risk of cardiovascular disease and uses small doses of cholesterol-lowering medication to keep this all-important risk factor in check.

Libby's physical examination was normal. Although her chest pain did not sound like typical heart pain (angina pectoris), an exercise stress thallium test was performed. Libby was able to exercise through stage 5 (out of 7) on the treadmill, suggesting that her symptoms were not due to heart problems. An upper gastrointestinal X ray (upper GI series) was performed. Libby swallowed liquid barium while radiologists observed the movement of this material through her esophagus, stomach, and part of her small intestines. The barium moved a little slower than expected down the esophagus into the stomach. The stomach was rather large and did not contract well. This resulted in barium remaining in the stomach for a long period of time before being expelled into the small intestines. Some of the liquid from the stomach was observed to flow back into the esophagus (called esophageal reflux, which often causes symptoms of heart burn), reaching the level of Libby's mid chest. Libby was treated with the medication cisapride to help stimulate her gastrointestinal tract, and an antacid pill (omeprazole). She felt better, and over the next few weeks, her symptoms of low blood sugar levels and chest discomfort disappeared.

Although it has not been proven, there is evidence that exercise and keeping blood sugar levels more tightly controlled can reduce some of the problems associated with diabetes (Table 5.4). Since the major cause of death among women (and men) is cardiovascular disease, we wanted to be more sure that Libby did not have heart disease. For women, probably until age 60, electrocardiogram exercise tests are not very helpful. That is why a nuclear medicine test (thallium scintigraphy in this case) or an exercise echocardiogram is a better diagnostic test to determine coronary heart disease. Fortunately, Libby had heartburn, or esophageal reflux, and delayed emptying of her stomach's contents into the small intestines, not heart disease. Because of this, her meals were not absorbed as fast as usual, and she was experiencing hypoglycemia symptoms because of the delay of food absorption. With the use of cisapride (Propulsid) prior to meals, her stomach was stimulated and moved the contents to the small intestine more rapidly. Libby then had fewer hypoglycemic episodes and less heartburn. Four years later, she is doing well.

Some Final Words of Advice

There are a number of benefits you can gain from regular exercise, including (1) better control of your blood sugar, (2) less need for insulin or pills to lower blood sugar (Type 1 or Type 2), (3) more effective insulin (either the insulin you inject, or the kind you make in your pancreas), (4) prevention or even reversal of diabetes (Type 2), (5) improved cardiovascular risk profile (Types 1 and 2) with lower blood pressure and an improved blood fat profile (cholesterol and triglycerides), and (6) probably fewer diabetes complications (Table 5.4). In addition, you will be fitter as well as feel and look better. That is not bad for two hours of exercise each week. You just can't buy that kind of benefit in a bottle.

Chapter 6

Exercise to Treat Abnormal Cholesterol Levels

There are many kinds of cholesterol, and like politicians, they are not all bad. Some are good (HDL_2 and HDL_3), some are not so good (VLDL), and one type is very harmful (LDL). In the United States, over 50 million people are at high risk for heart and blood vessel disease because of the cholesterol in their bloodstream. Millions more are at risk because of borderline levels. Many lives and billions of dollars in disability and medical costs can be saved with effective treatment. But treatment does not necessarily mean using drugs. Exercise can rearrange your cholesterol levels to reduce your chance of heart attack and stroke. In fact, more than half of those at risk can be treated without any medication.

To illustrate the link between exercise and cholesterol, we provide you with three of our own clinical cases. You may want to refer to Table 6.1, which lists risk levels for triglyceride levels and the major types of cholesterol levels. Ask your health care provider about your levels and use the table to check your personal risk for heart and blood vessel disease.

Cholesterol Ratios

It is not just the levels of LDL and HDL that are important. The balance between the amounts of each type of cholesterol, found by dividing your total amount of cholesterol by your amount of HDL cholesterol, can help determine your risk. The lower the ratio, the better. A ratio of 4.5/1 is the average risk, while a ratio of 3/1 reduces your chance of coronary heart disease by approximately half. As the balance

TABLE 6.1 **Cholesterol Risk**

Risk Level	Total Cholesterol (mg/dL)	LDL Cholesterol (mg/dL)	HDL Cholesterol (mg/dL)	Triglycerides (mg/dL)
High risk	Over 245	Over 190	Below 35	Over 1,000
Moderate risk	221–245	160–190	36–44	400–1,000
Mild risk	201–220	130–159	45–54	250–399
Average risk	180–200	100–129	55–65	150–249
Low risk	Below 180	Below 100	Over 65	Below 150

between total cholesterol and HDL cholesterol climbs to 7, the risk doubles.

Meagan is a 26-year-old assistant manager of a local exercise facility. She came to the Human Performance Laboratory to check her body fat and cholesterol levels. After winning a number of local and regional contests, Meagan's desire was to become a professional bodybuilder. Each day she exercised with heavy doses of aerobics and hours of pumping iron. Standing 5 feet, 9 inches tall and weighing 175 pounds, she appeared extremely fit and muscular. Although her muscle size was large, there were no signs of masculinization (no facial hair, balding, or deep voice).

Because she was preparing for an upcoming bodybuilding contest, her diet was severely restricted. Meagan was feeling irritable and fatigued on only 600 calories per day. Her diet was designed to strip her body of unwanted fat so she could "show off" her muscles. Meagan avoided any food that contained fat. Protein powder shakes, amino acid tablets, and dry fruit were the main menu items.

After being weighed under water, she was happy to learn that her body fat measured 6 percent (normal for a woman is 20 to 25 percent body fat). But her laboratory results revealed another story. Despite a total cholesterol level in the low-risk range of 160 mg/dL, and an LDL cholesterol level in the average-risk category (128 mg/dL), Meagan's HDL cholesterol level was terrible at only 7 mg/dL. This was the lowest (and worst) value we had ever seen. Her ratio of total to HDL cholesterol was off the scale at almost 23!

So despite her low-fat diet, high volume of exercise, and being the "top gun" in the local bodybuilding world, Meagan's cardiovascular risk was definitely in the danger zone. Her family history did not reveal any cardiovascular disease or cholesterol problems, and she said her health was excellent. We decided to ask Meagan a few more questions that might tell us why her HDL level was so low.

Nearly all forms of exercise, including bodybuilding and other types of weight lifting will improve cholesterol levels. When we saw the low HDL level, we thought it might be a laboratory error. However, we asked Meagan about any drugs she was using. Meagan had great cholesterol levels at one time, but these levels all but vanished as she began to use anabolic steroids to reshape her body. Anabolic steroids are copies of the male hormone testosterone, and these can wipe out HDL cholesterol when used at very high doses, despite all the hard work athletes may do. Unfortunately, Meagan had only the veneer of wellness. Her risk for cardiovascular disease was very high.

High-Risk Cholesterol

Phil is 44 years old and always feels tired. But you wouldn't think it by his travel schedule and his outstanding work as a senior strategist for a high-tech software company. Traveling around the world, he felt at home while flying at 30,000 feet. In fact, he averaged little more than one week at his residence during most months of the year. Married to his third wife, Phil had a daughter and an adopted son. Between work and family, there seemed to be little time for exercise or other recreational activities.

Phil's medical history revealed that he had high blood pressure, treated with a number of medications over the past few years. He complained that each medication made him feel worse than the last. His diet was healthy—he limited his intake of high-fat foods such as red meat, cheese, and eggs.

Now, despite his diet, Phil needed to add his high cholesterol level to his high blood pressure as risks for heart and blood vessel disease. Phil's total cholesterol measured 278 mg/dL, with LDL cholesterol of 162 mg/dL, and HDL cholesterol of 54 mg/dL. His triglyceride level was mildly elevated at 260 mg/dL. Despite a lean appearance in his suit, Phil's body fat measured 25 percent (normal for an adult man is 12 to 18 percent).

Phil was placed on a very low fat (less than 20 percent of his calories were from fat) and a low-salt (2 grams of sodium) diet. After four weeks, he complained that his diet was very low in taste, too. His blood pressure remained elevated, and follow-up tests of his cholesterol and triglyceride levels were not much better.

Since he was not planning to leave the area for the next six weeks, Phil decided to join the exercise clinic at the hospital and began aerobics and stationary cycling. After a physical examination and screening treadmill electrocardiogram, he found his exercise heart rate range to be 130 to 160 beats per minute. Using his electronic daily planner as a guide, he began to exercise four days each week for 45 minutes per session. We planned to recheck his lipoprotein levels in about three months, if he continued his routine.

Phil's story is really quite common. He was able to change his diet and began to alter his lifestyle by coming to the exercise clinic. Not being one who would be content with moderate exercise, he competed in triathalons (contests involving swimming, biking, and running) and went to fitness camps in the summer. Adding exercise to his lifestyle boosted the effect of his low-fat diet. Unfortunately, he would often overdo his training, which resulted in various injuries. However, Phil was inventive and switched from one type of exercise, such as running, to swimming when this occured. His HDL cholesterol level climbed to over 60 mg/dL, and his LDL cholesterol decreased. Ten years later, he continues to exercise, eat well . . . and travel.

Can Great Cholesterol Levels Become Better?

With a total cholesterol level of 162 mg/dL, HDL cholesterol of 51 mg/dL, and LDL cholesterol of 107 mg/dL, Sandi might ruin the study. Her levels just were too good.

Sandi, Dr. Goldberg's sister-in-law, was entered into our study at the insistence of her sister (Dr. Goldberg's wife, Marsha). Until 18 months ago, when she started studying for her master's degree, Sandi had trained regularly with her college dance troupe. Now with her degree in cultural anthropology, she moved to the big city without a job, a place to stay, or a social life. Her sister believed that being a part of a diverse group of study subjects, all trying to become fit, would be the perfect treatment for her sister. The problem was that Sandi's cholesterol already looked great! If her cholesterol was too good, it might not improve, no matter what she did.

We were beginning a study of exercise and cholesterol that, unlike many of the other exercise studies that used aerobic exercise, involved only weight lifting. In 1982, using strength training to improve your health was heresy to the exercise science world. Exercise was aerobics, and *only* aerobics (for example, jogging, cycling, and aerobic dance). Weight lifting was not considered to be a type of physical activity that made you healthier. Furthermore, this was a heavy, strength-building training program. If you could lift a weight eight times or more, we slapped on another 10 pounds.

Sandi brought other intangibles to the study besides her great lipid levels. She became the cheerleader in the group. She worked hard and encouraged others as she pumped iron, going from weight station to weight station, stopping occasionally to view a new muscular bulge in her arms and legs. If Sandi missed a workout, Dr. Goldberg became her personal trainer at the local Jewish Community Center on the weekend. She occasionally worked out extra times at the community center, sometimes with the Portland Trailblazer basketball team. She began to develop a reputation as "the superwoman."

Although her blood fat levels were superb, Sandi's cholesterol levels improved even further. Her HDL cholesterol level increased, and her triglyceride and LDL cholesterol levels dropped to record lows. Was our study published? It can be found in the Olympic edition of the *Journal of the American Medical Association* (1984). Although not everyone will find true love and happiness by entering into an exercise study, it worked for Sandi. First, she met a local television producer who was also in the study. He gave her a job at the station so she could move out of the guest bedroom at the Goldberg's house. Then, while making up a missed training session, under the watchful eye of her brother-in-law, she met a very handsome (we had to say it) man who was impressed with the amount of weight she could lift. They spoke, dated, became engaged, and after a "heavy courtship," married. Today they have two lovely children. Sandi continues to train every day and was even featured in the state's major newspaper for her personal weight-lifting program. Dr. Goldberg still continues to take credit for her happiness.

What Is Fat?

In general, when people talk about fat, they are speaking of any substance that is made of small molecules called *fatty acids*. When

Fat is a very concentrated source of energy. It has over twice the number of calories (9 calories/gram) as carbohydrates or protein (each 4 calories/gram). So a pound of fat (3,500 calories) has more than twice the calories of 2 pounds of sugar or 2 pounds of protein.

three fatty acids are linked to a molecule called *glycerol,* a triglyceride (*tri* = three fatty acids, glycerol = *glyceride*) is formed. Triglycerides often are made from the fats we eat or can be manufactured in our bodies from other food sources, such as carbohydrates. Triglycerides are the main storage form of fat and energy in our body, and these stores can provide fuel for up to 100 hours of continuous exercise. Also, body fat is needed for production of certain hormones, and it cushions our organs and stores reserves of vitamins A, D, E, and K.

What Is Cholesterol?

Although not strictly a fat, cholesterol is a waxy substance that travels in the company of triglycerides and other fats. But remember, don't judge all cholesterol just by the company it keeps. Our bodies make and need some cholesterol, as do all other four-limbed animals. Cholesterol is an essential part of our cells' membranes. Furthermore, cholesterol is the backbone for steroid hormones (such as estrogen and testosterone) and vitamin D and is an essential ingredient of our liver's bile, which helps us digest the fat we eat. So, our body needs cholesterol. Otherwise we have no sex hormones and our cells fall apart. Unfortunately, too much cholesterol can have disastrous effects. Cholesterol is a major ingredient in the fatty deposits that form on the walls of our arteries, clogging blood flow to our heart, brain, muscles, and other tissues.

What Are Lipoproteins?

Good question. No, make that a great question. When scientists discuss triglyceride and cholesterol levels, they often speak of them together as lipoproteins. In the same way oil and water do not mix, triglycerides and cholesterol cannot simply dissolve in our blood. Because of this, triglycerides and cholesterol require a special chemical transporter. The transporter is a combination of lipids (fats) and unique proteins called apoproteins. Thus the term *lipoprotein* is derived from the word *lipid* (or *lipo*) and the word *protein.*

The Good, the Bad, and the Ugly

Lipoproteins, or blood fats, take several forms. The main substances are (1) chylomicrons, (2) HDL (high-density lipoprotein) cholesterol, (3) VLDL (very low density lipoprotein), and (4) LDL (low-density lipoprotein) cholesterol.

When people mention their cholesterol level, they are usually speaking of total cholesterol. Your total cholesterol is a combination of all the different types of cholesterol, the good, the bad, and the . . . well you get the picture.

Chylomicrons

Chylomicrons (pronounced ky-low-my-krons) come from the fats we eat. Because fats are not well absorbed in their natural state, they need to be converted (or morphed) into a more absorbable substance. As fat passes from the stomach into our small intestines, the enzymatic action of our pancreatic juices and bile from our liver and gall bladder create chylomicrons by rearranging these fat molecules and improving digestion.

Chylomicrons contain mostly triglycerides. There are some people with abnormal chylomicron production, based on genetic problems. They are able to produce chylomicrons but are unable to also break them down. However, for most of us, the enzyme *lipoprotein lipase* breaks down chylomicrons. This enzyme slices off the fatty acids from the glycerol molecule; then we can use the fatty acids for energy or store them in our fat cells.

HDL Cholesterol

There are two major forms of HDL cholesterol, referred to as HDL_2 and HDL_3. Both forms protect us against cardiovascular disease. Most laboratories combine HDL_2 and HDL_3 counts and refer to the total as just HDL cholesterol.

HDL travels around in your bloodstream, sucking up cholesterol, much like a biological vacuum cleaner. HDL carries waxy cholesterol away from fatty deposits on your arteries, to be broken down in the liver. The higher your HDL cholesterol level, the better the cleaning job and the lower your risk of heart and blood vessel disease. To help you remember what is good for you, just remember that you want your *high*-density lipoprotein cholesterol to be *high*. The higher, the better.

VLDL Cholesterol

Excess triglycerides in the blood stream are linked to coronary heart disease. High levels can be caused by genetic abnormalities, excessive fat intake, or uncontrolled metabolic problems such as diabetes.

VLDL cholesterol contains mainly triglycerides, just like chylomicrons. VLDL can be formed by breaking up chylomicrons or can be manufactured by your liver. Then these triglyceride-loaded particles can be either transported to the rest of the body and used as energy, or stored in your thighs, waist, derriere, and other fat depots. Although high VLDL levels are related to coronary heart disease, they are not as damaging as LDL cholesterol. When VLDL (or chylomicron) levels increase, high triglyceride levels result and your HDL cholesterol level drops. This can compound the harm of a high VLDL cholesterol level.

LDL Cholesterol

LDL cholesterol is known as the "bad" cholesterol. Picture a molecule wearing a black cowboy hat, squeezing your arteries with black gloves, and depositing globs of yellow fat plaques. LDL cholesterol is a powerful risk factor for cardiovascular disease. For those without diseased blood vessels, reducing LDL cholesterol levels below 110 mg/dL will probably improve your ability to avoid heart disease. However, if you have coronary heart disease, it is recommended that your LDL-cholesterol be lower than 100 mg/dL. At this level, cholesterol plaques begin to dissolve, and arteries become unobstructed. You want your low-density lipoprotein cholesterol level to be low. The lower, the better.

Exercise and Cholesterol Levels

Despite medical breakthroughs, during the last 60 to 75 years Americans have exercised less, and this has reduced our ability to live longer, healthier lives. If lack of exercise can be likened to a major weapon directed at our health, then surely cholesterol is one of the most harmful bullets. The cholesterol circulating in your blood is a combination of LDL, VLDL, and HDL cholesterols. So you always have both good and bad cholesterol, and the main portion of the total cholesterol is LDL cholesterol. High total cholesterol levels are strongly associated with cardiovascular disease, and cardiovascular disease is the number-one killer in the United States, as well as in most other industrialized countries.

As you have learned, triglycerides are another risk factor for coronary heart disease because they assist in the build-up of harmful fatty plaques and reduce the sucking power of our body's vacuum-cleaning (HDL) cholesterol. In addition, very high triglyceride levels (over 1,000 mg/dL) can damage your pancreas and cause your liver to swell.

Improving your blood cholesterol levels will reduce your risk of heart and blood vessel disease and will prolong your life. Predictions from long-term studies suggest that over 60 percent of coronary heart disease can be prevented by lowering the total cholesterol level just 20 percent, or LDL cholesterol by 30 percent. In addition as you become more fit, your physical stresses will be easier to manage, and you will be better able to reduce your emotional stress as well. So life just might seem a whole lot easier.

Reducing your total cholesterol level by just 3 percent will lower your chance of developing coronary heart disease by 15 percent.

What Kind of Treatment Improves Cholesterol Levels?

Drugs that lower cholesterol and triglyceride levels can be very effective therapy, but they are often quite expensive. For example, the most commonly used medicines, namely the 3-hydroxy-3-methylglutaryl coenzyme A (HMG-CoA) reductase inhibitors, also called statins, can cost about $420 to $2,640 per year, depending on the dose you need (Table 6.2), and you may not be lucky enough to have your insurance pay for your medication. So, while your neighbor takes his family to Disneyland, you stay at home to earn enough money to pay for your cholesterol-lowering drugs.

The medications listed in Table 6.2 are some of the major cholesterol- and triglyceride-reducing drug therapies. In addition, the vitamin niacin, in the form of nicotinic acid, can be used. Nicotinic acid, sold over-the-counter, lowers triglyceride and LDL cholesterol levels and raises HDL cholesterol levels. Although effective, you must take at least

TABLE 6.2 **Drugs That Improve Lipoprotein Levels**			
Generic Name (Trade Name)	**Starting Daily Dose (Approximate)**	**What It Does**	**Cost for 30 Days (Approximate)**
Atrovastatin (Lipitor)	10 mg	Greatly lowers LDL, raises HDL, and decreases triglycerides	$55.00
Cholestyramine (Questran, Prevalite)	8 grams (2 scoops)	Greatly lowers LDL	$35.00
Fenofibrate (TriCor)	67 mg	Greatly lowers triglycerides and LDL; raises HDL	$26.00
Fluvastatin (Lescol)	20 mg	Modestly lowers LDL and raises HDL	$37.00
Gemfibrozil (Lopid)	1,200 mg	Greatly lowers triglycerides and slightly raises HDL	$55.00
Lovastatin (Mevacor)	20 mg	Greatly lowers LDL, raises HDL, and slightly reduces triglycerides	$67.50
Pravastatin (Pravachol)	20 mg	Greatly lowers LDL, raises HDL, and slightly reduces triglycerides	$59.00
Simvastatin (Zocor)	10 mg	Greatly lowers LDL, raises HDL, and slightly reduces triglycerides	$61.00
Cerivastatin (Baycol)	0.3 mg	Greatly lowers LDL, raises HDL, and slightly lowers triglycerides	$45.00

400 mg each day to have a positive result. Typically, the dose is slowly increased to about 1.5 to 3 grams each day. At these dosages, nicotinic acid often causes uncomfortable flushing and gastrointestinal upset, and some people develop gout, a very painful form of arthritis. Also, because high doses of niacin can increase blood sugar levels, it should be used with caution if you have diabetes. Please note that nicotinamide, another form of the vitamin, does not lower cholesterol levels. A newer prescription formulation, Niaspan, is an extended-release niacin tablet. The dose of Niaspan is slowly increased over a three-month period. Although it produces fewer gastrointestinal and flushing symptoms, it is more expensive than over-the-counter nicotinic acid.

Most lipoprotein-lowering drugs have few side effects. Medications that treat only very high triglyceride levels may cause gall bladder problems. However, muscle weakness and abnormal liver enzyme levels can result from many of these drugs. So, make sure your health care provider checks your liver enzymes if you are using these drugs. Also, these medications can interact with other drugs you may be taking.

Since many of us have more than one health care provider but just one body, it is important to give each provider a list of your medications before taking a new drug.

Another group of cholesterol modifiers consists of substances made by plants, called phytosterols and stanols. Although the molecules resemble cholesterol, humans cannot absorb them very well. When added to our diet, phytosterols and stanols interfere with our ability to absorb cholesterol. In a Finnish study, adding these substances to margarine-like spreads lowered LDL cholesterol levels by 10 percent. Likewise, adding psyllium seed or bran to your diet can lower LDL cholesterol levels by about 10 percent.

Other ways to improve your cholesterol levels include eating large amounts of fruits, vegetables, and whole grain foods, lowering your total amount of body fat, and avoiding smoking and second-hand smoke.

Estrogen and Cholesterol

Female hormones (estrogens) are one of the reasons that women are temporarily protected from heart disease and are typically about 10 years older than men when coronary disease strikes. After menopause, women can use estrogen or estrogen-like hormones to reduce LDL cholesterol and increase HDL cholesterol levels. These cholesterol levels usually change in the healthy direction by 15 percent each. Estrogen replacement therapy reduces the risk of heart disease by about 50 percent. A newer medication, raloxifene, has estrogen-like effects on bones and cholesterol levels. However, when tested in experimental animals, raloxifene was ineffective at reducing coronary artery obstruction when compared with estrogen.

Different Fats in Food

Although all fats contain the same amount of calories (9 calories for each gram), they are not all the same with regard to our health (Table 6.3). Most fats can be categorized as either saturated or unsaturated fats, based on their chemical structure. As a general rule, saturated fats are

TABLE 6.3 **The Lowdown on Fats**

Type of Fat	Where Found	What It Does
Saturated	Worst is palmitic acid; most found in animal fat, also in coconut and palm oil	Raises total and LDL cholesterol; may cause certain cancers
Polyunsaturated	Vegetable oils, such as safflower sunflower, soybean, and corn	In small amounts it lowers LDL cholesterol; In high amounts that cause weight gain, it can decrease HDL and raise LDL cholesterol
Monounsaturated*	Oils such as olive, canola, peanut; also in peanuts, avocado, olives, pecans	Lowers LDL cholesterol
Omega-3 fatty acids	Fish oil and canola oil	Lowers triglycerides; also may reduce heart disease by lowering stickiness of platelets to reduce chance of blood clots

*When monounsaturated fats are hydrogenated (hardened) into more solid forms, such as margarine, they lose their cholesterol-lowering effect and are not much better than butter.

unhealthy and unsaturated fats are not unhealthy. In general, you can tell if a fat is saturated or unsaturated by how it appears at room temperature. Unsaturated fats are usually liquid, while saturated fats are solid at 70 degrees fahrenheit. Typically, the harder the fat, the more saturated it is. Butter, the animal product, is mainly saturated fat.

What is important to know is that meat from animals with four legs, many dairy products, and animal organs, even chicken liver, contain very high amounts of saturated fat. Eating these fats leads to high blood pressure, certain types of cancer, and heart and blood vessel diseases.

Vegetable Fats

Just because a fat is from vegetable sources does not mean it is healthy, especially when we start messing around with Mother Nature. By chemically changing a fat's structure, we can create problems. For instance, hardening liquid vegetable oil to form stick margarine causes it to lose much of its unsaturated benefits. The reason stick margarine becomes more unhealthy is the process called hydrogenation. In this procedure, by-products called trans fatty acids are made. Trans fatty acids lower your good, HDL cholesterol level and raise your unhealthy, LDL cholesterol level, just like saturated fat. So, as liquid vegetable oil turns into a substance that looks like a stick of butter, it becomes almost as unhealthy as butter.

The bottom line is that just because a margarine label says the product is low in cholesterol and saturated fat, that does not mean it is a healthy product. When fat is solid at room temperature, it is best to avoid it!

The Best Edible Fats

Not all fats are bad. But, animals (including us) do not make some of the healthier, less-saturated fats. Unlike their saturated cousins, mono-unsaturated and polyunsaturated fats are healthy. Also, there are certain fatty acids we need, but cannot make, and therefore we need to eat those fatty acids that are essential to our health.

Some fats contain omega-3 and omega-6 fatty acids, and these substances actually lower LDL cholesterol levels. Omega-3 fatty acids, found in fish, can reduce triglyceride levels (as long as the fish is not deep fried in animal fat or fat with high levels of trans fatty acids, such as hard margarine). Table 6.3 lists various types of fats, where they are found, and the effects of diets that are high in each fat.

The amount of cholesterol you eat is less important than the amount of saturated fat in your diet. Most dietary cholesterol comes from egg yolks, dairy products, and red meat. We recommend eating less than 300 mg of cholesterol each day. If you have a high LDL cholesterol level, limit your intake to 200 mg per day.

Why Is My Cholesterol Different From Yours?

Our blood fat levels are controlled by many factors: what we eat, the levels of male and female hormones, genetic traits, smoking habits (lowers HDL cholesterol), our weight and percentage of body fat, the drugs we take, and the amount of exercise we get. The only factor we can't change, no matter how hard we try, is our heredity. All the others can be altered by the choices we make.

Women have the benefit of estrogen, which increases HDL cholesterol levels and may be responsible for the fact that women live approximately seven years longer than men. Smoking cigarettes lowers

HDL cholesterol levels, which is one reason it is one of the major risk factors for heart disease. Certain drugs can worsen our cholesterol and triglyceride levels, especially diuretics (water pills) and certain blood pressure and heart medications called beta blockers. Small amounts of alcohol (one to two drinks a day) may raise HDL cholesterol levels; however, higher amounts will increase triglyceride levels. In our society, alcohol abuse does much more harm to our health than can be offset by its ability to raise HDL cholesterol levels a few points.

Our Heredity and Our Blood Fats

We might not like it, but our heredity—the genes that make us unique beings—has a giant impact on our cholesterol and triglyceride levels. Some people have familial cholesterol and triglyceride abnormalities that, without treatment, can shorten lifespans and create rapidly progressive disease. It is important for anyone whose father, mother, or close relative had heart or blood vessel disease before age 50, to see his or her health care provider to measure cholesterol and triglyceride levels.

Breaking Down Cholesterol and Triglycerides

For greater health, we want our body to break down LDL cholesterol, chylomicrons, and VLDL (our main triglyceride particles) and create more HDL cholesterol "vacuum cleaners." Although we often blame our shortcomings on heredity, we can take the bull by the horns (rather than eat the steer) and lower LDL cholesterol and triglyceride levels by making wise dietary choices (especially how much and what kind of fat we eat) and supercharging our fat-busting enzymes by losing excess body fat and getting regular exercise. The level of fat-metabolizing enzymes in your body depends, in part, on the amount and type of exercise you do.

What to Eat?

As far as our blood fat levels are concerned, highly saturated fats will increase LDL cholesterol levels by blocking our liver's ability to break up the LDL molecules. By limiting saturated fat or the amount of cholesterol in our food, our liver becomes more effective at eliminating this harmful form of cholesterol. Eating foods high in polyunsaturated fats can help lower LDL cholesterol levels. Monosaturated fats and those fats that contain omega-3 fatty acids can be helpful, especially when they take the place of saturated fats in our diet.

The Heart-Healthy Diet

Although we need fat to survive, particularly the essential fatty acids mentioned earlier, it is important to limit our fat intake, no matter what kind of fat it is. For those without abnormal cholesterol levels, keep the total calories from fat below 30 percent and total daily cholesterol intake to less than 300 mg. That's easy to remember: below 30 and 300. If you have problems with cholesterol, we recommend reducing total fat intake to about 20 percent of total calories and limiting the cholesterol in your diet to less than 200 mg each day. Table 6.4 lists some recommended diet therapies for high cholesterol levels.

By making simple food choices, you can lower your very bad cholesterol. Try doing the following:

TABLE 6.4	**Cholesterol-Lowering Diets (amounts/day)**		
Nutrient	**Recommended for Everyone**	**Higher Risk**	**Mediterranean**
Total fat (percentage of total calories)	30%	20%	Less than 40%
Saturated fat (percentage of total calories)	About 10 %	About 5%	About 10%
Polyunsaturated fat (percentage of total calories)	About 10%	About 10%	About 10%
Monounsaturated fat (percentage of total calories)	About 10%	About 10%	About 20%
Cholesterol	300 mg or less	200 mg or less	300 mg or less
Carbohydrates (percentage of total calories)	About 55%	About 60%	About 45%
Protein (percentage of total calories)	About 15%	About 15%	About 15%

- Select fish or skinned turkey and chicken, instead of red meat
- Use skim milk instead of the types with 2 percent or greater fat content
- Choose canola or olive oil for cooking
- Limit egg yolks to four or fewer each week
- Eat plenty of fresh vegetables and fruits
- Avoid desserts with a high fat content
- Reduce alcohol consumption to one or two drinks each day
- Don't eat unless you are hungry and stop eating when you are not hungry

If you are eating the typical American diet, which is not a healthy one, you can expect to reduce your cholesterol level by following any one of the diets found in Table 6.4, with the listing of each diet's major nutrient amounts.

If your total cholesterol level is 240 mg/dL, you will lower it by about 11 mg/dL with the general recommended diet and 20 mg/dL with the higher-risk diet. If your LDL cholesterol is 160 mg/dL, the general recommended diet will drop your LDL level by about 7 mg/dL, while the high-risk diet will drop it by a little more than 12 mg/dL. If you lost weight, your cholesterol and LDL levels will drop even further. The Mediterranean diet is similar to the recommended diet in changing your LDL cholesterol level. However, it has an advantage of not reducing your HDL cholesterol, a problem that can occur when you reduce fat and increase carbohydrates. However, all diets work best when you are at your optimum weight (also see Chapter 7).

Fat is essential to our health. Fat contains vitamins A, D, E, and K. It is part of our cell membranes and is needed to form certain hormones.

Your Fat-Busting Enzymes

Certain types of enzymes control our body's cholesterol and triglyceride levels. These enzymes can be changed by drugs, your body fat and muscle mass, and whether you exercise.

One enzyme, named lipoprotein lipase, also known as LPL, is located in the walls of our blood vessels and in our heart, fat stores, and muscles. This enzyme breaks down triglycerides. Low levels of LPL are associated with increased cardiovascular disease. So, higher LPL levels are good, and things that stimulate LPL action will help us avoid coronary heart disease.

Another enzyme, hepatic lipase (HL), breaks down HDL cholesterol, but in the process converts some of it to harmful LDL cholesterol. The higher our HL enzyme level, the lower our HDL cholesterol level, which increases the risk of developing heart disease.

A third important enzyme, with the very long name of lecithin cholesterol acyl transferase, is better known as LCAT. Although it sounds to us like a piece of heavy machinery that moves dirt ("Hey, get that LCAT over here to clear this section of land!"), it actually grabs onto cholesterol, cleaning it off of artery walls, in a way that is similar to the powerful sucking of a professional-quality vacuum cleaner.

Enzyme Changes and Exercise

Production of the enzymes that control our blood fat levels can be changed by exercise. LPL, the enzyme that breaks down triglycerides and increases HDL cholesterol levels, has been found in greater quantity among aerobic exercisers. Its effects are increased after just one exercise session. Also, losing body fat will increase the action of LPL.

Hepatic lipase (HL) is the enzyme that clears out our good HDL cholesterol and breaks it down. Endurance exercise tends to increase the amount of HDL cholesterol by reducing the activity of HL. One study found that HL action was lowered among middle-aged men after 15 weeks of exercise, although not all studies have found similar results. Likewise, the amount of LCAT, the enzyme that takes up cholesterol from the artery walls, can be increased by exercise. Not everyone will improve his or her enzyme function with exercise, likely due to individual differences. Similarly, not all drugs affect us in the same way, which is why we have so many different medications for the same medical problem. However, for many people, exercise can generate more enzyme activity and improve our blood fat levels.

Running Down Cholesterol and Triglycerides

In the mid 1970s, researchers at Stanford looked at the blood fat profiles of runners and of inactive men. They found that the amounts of protective HDL cholesterol were higher in the joggers, while triglyceride levels were significantly lower. Over the next few years, 66 studies concerned with the effect of exercise on cholesterol were published by researchers. When these programs were bundled together and analyzed, total cholesterol levels were lowered an average of 10 mg/dL, while triglycerides were reduced by an average of 16 mg/dL. When the researchers looked at the bad (LDL) and good (HDL) cholesterol, they found that LDL cholesterol was lowered even more, and HDL cholesterol was raised. This was great news. Exercise changed all the major blood fat levels—and all in the right direction.

Cutting Cholesterol with Weight Lifting

By the early 1980s, it was becoming more clear that aerobic training improved cholesterol levels and burned up triglycerides, too. But what about pumping iron? Most scientists thought lifting weights was for those who wanted to look good, rather than be healthy, but they were wrong.

As we described earlier in this chapter, weight lifting, or any kind of resistance exercise using springs, bands, or air pressure, can change cholesterol levels. In several studies, including our own publication in the *Journal of the American Medical Association,* strength training lowered LDL cholesterol levels and improved the ratio of good (HDL) to total cholesterol levels. We found these benefits occured among both men and women after just 16 weeks of exercise. In our program, participants worked out three times each week, lifting weights for approximately 45 minutes to 1 hour. Our study participants used moderately heavy weights. If they could lift a weight 8 times (upper body) or 12 times (lower body), the amount of weight was increased by about 10 pounds (upper body) or 20 pounds (lower body). Altogether, our subjects used eight different exercises, with a minimum of three or four sets of three to eight repetitions per exercise (Table 6.5).

Why Diet If I Exercise?

Although this book is about exercise, we can't emphasize enough the importance of your diet. We all splurge and eat foods that are loaded with fats, but this can't be the rule. You can magnify the benefits of

TABLE 6.5 **Weight-Lifting Exercises to Change Cholesterol**		
	Sets	**Reps**
Upper Body Exercises		
Bench press	4	3–8
Latissimus pull	3	3–8
Shoulder press	3	3–8
Arm curl	3	3–8
Rows	3	3–8
Lower Body Exercises		
Leg press	4	6–12
Leg extension	3	6–12
Leg curl	3	6–12

your workouts by making wise food choices. On the other hand, you can ruin all your hard work by poor food selections. For example, rewarding yourself for a workout by eating a typical cheeseburger will add more calories to your body than you would use on a five-mile run. In addition, you will be pummeling your body with high doses of saturated fat from the red meat and cheese.

Because we did not emphasize the importance of not changing his diet to Dave, one of our study subjects, he proceeded to eat much more fat that he did prior to training. When we asked Dave why, he said, "Since exercise will lower my cholesterol, I should be able to eat more ice cream and other desserts, without having my cholesterol increase." Although Dave's cholesterol level did decrease, the benefits of exercise were not as dramatic as they could have been.

Do I Still Need to Exercise If I Change My Diet?

Don't think that changing your diet is all you need. It is not. We base this on our own clinical experience plus volumes of research. In a 1998 study reported in the *New England Journal of Medicine*, researchers followed nearly 400 men and women who had levels of LDL cholesterol between 125 mg/dL and 210 mg/dL Exercise training was in the form of brisk walking or jogging 10 miles each week. Participants were divided into four groups:

Group 1. Diet without exercise
Group 2. No special diet, but regular exercise
Group 3. Diet plus regular exercise
Group 4. No special diet and no exercise

The diet was very low in cholesterol and saturated fat. Study subjects were observed for one year. What were the results?

All exercisers improved their fitness, whether they dieted or not.
Dieters who lowered fat intake from 30 percent to 22 percent of total calories lost about 7.5 pounds, whether they exercised or not.
Only dieters who exercised lowered their LDL cholesterol levels (by about 11 percent).

The authors of this study concluded that lowering fat intake from 30 percent to 22 percent of total calories lowers cholesterol only when you exercise.

Adding exercise to a diet low in saturated fat doubles the diet's cholesterol-lowering effect.

However, it is important for us to remember that the typical American diet is so high in fat that when we eat 30 percent of our calories from fat, most of us will dramatically improve our cholesterol and triglyceride levels. Either a diet or exercise alone can improve your blood fat levels. But when exercise and diet are combined, they become a potent antidote for abnormal cholesterol levels.

How Much Exercise Do I Need?

Improving cholesterol and triglyceride levels usually requires a large dose of exercise. For instance, you can lower your blood pressure with 30 minutes of moderate walking, three times each week. However, more exercise is needed for cholesterol manipulation. If you are inactive and want to improve your cholesterol and triglyceride levels, you need to exercise the equivalent of 8 to 10 miles of jogging or brisk walking each week. The more miles you log, the higher your HDL cholesterol level can climb. Also, lowering the amount of fat in your diet will add to these cholesterol and triglyceride benefits. If you want to lower your LDL cholesterol by lifting weights, you need to work out for 45 to 60 minutes, three times each week. The successful programs are shown in Tables 6.5 and 6.6.

How Long Will It Take to See Reduced Cholesterol Levels?

Don't despair if you fail to see improved cholesterol levels during the first few weeks of training. You will begin to feel better, and your endurance will improve even before you see enzyme and blood chemistry changes. After 12 weeks of aerobic exercise, about 50 percent of regular exercisers will have increased their HDL cholesterol levels. But, it can take more than 6 months to achieve cholesterol improvements from aerobic training, even when you are exercising four to five times each week. This is especially true when there is no accompanying

---

TABLE 6.6   **Formula for Exercise**

Type of Exercise
Aerobics or weightlifting (your choice)
Aerobics more effective at raising HDL cholesterol
Weight lifting more effective at lowering LDL cholesterol

Intensity (how hard)
75 to 85 percent of maximal heart rate, or perceived exertion level 3 to 4 (out of 10) for aerobics
For weight lifting, check out Chapter 12

Duration (how long)
20 minutes initially, increasing to 45 to 60 minutes

Frequency (how often)
At least four times each week for aerobics
At least three times each week for weight lifting

weight loss. Remember, you are changing your lifestyle to feel better and have a longer and healthier life. That takes time.

Besides changing your cholesterol and triglyceride levels, other important changes will occur, such as lowering your blood pressure (see Chapter 8), strengthening your bones (see Chapter 3), and keeping fat pounds from accumulating around your waist (see Chapter 7).

Power Boosting the Effects of Exercise

There are a number of ways to boost the cholesterol and triglyceride changes that will occur with exercise (Table 6.7). As you have learned, lowering the amount of fat in your diet can nearly double the effect of exercise alone. Getting close to 20 percent of calories from fat may be optimal for people who are at high risk. However, if you eat fat that is rich in omega-3 fatty acids, you can lower triglyceride levels even more. Monounsaturated fatty acids, found in high amounts in the Mediterranean diet (Table 6.4), can lower LDL cholesterol levels. In those countries with the highest monosaturated fat intake, such as Italy and Greece, coronary heart disease is very low.

In addition to all the other harmful effects smoking has, it also lowers HDL cholesterol levels. If you smoke, stop. You will become fitter, and your HDL cholesterol level can rise even higher with physical activity. In other words, you will be smokin', rather than be a smoker.

TABLE 6.7   Treating High Cholesterol and Triglyceride Levels without Drugs

- Exercise
- Eat a diet low in saturated fat
- Use mono- and polyunsaturated fats
- Keep cholesterol intake below 300 mg per day
- Don't smoke
- Lose excess body fat
- Use estrogens (postmenopausal women only)
- Stop certain medications when possible (beta blockers, diuretics)

If you are overweight, weight loss will enhance the effect of your exercise on cholesterol and triglyceride levels. This means your triglyceride and LDL cholesterol levels can be lowered, and your HDL cholesterol level will increase. Just losing 5 to 10 pounds of fat can dramatically lower LDL and raise HDL levels.

Diuretics (water pills) or beta blockers such as propranolol, atenolol, or metoprolol can worsen cholesterol and triglyceride levels. Switching to another type of medication, such as ACE inhibitors or angiotensin II blockers, can help boost the effects of your exercise.

Exercise literally supercharges the metabolic transformation of your blood fats. Although it may take a few months to show up on laboratory reports, these changes can lead to a longer and healthier life.

Chapter 7

Exercise to Lose Weight

Marta is a 32-year-old nurse, and when first examined almost 18 months ago, she weighed 247 pounds and stood 5 feet, 10 inches tall. Her calculated BMI was 35 (body mass index = weight ÷ height^2 [see Tables 7.2 and 7.3]), and a BMI more than 30 is considered unhealthy. Other than being overweight, she felt well. When asked about her family, she said that both her parents were "very overweight." She had been chubby as a child and weighed 165 pounds at her high school graduation. Marta has gained about 5 pounds a year since then, plus adding more with each of her two pregnancies. Many attempts at weight loss resulted in a drop of 10 to 15 pounds, but she quickly regained the weight, becoming more frustrated with each attempt. She has been to Weight Watchers and Jenny Craig and knows more about nutrition than many physicians.

Her most recent diet began a few weeks ago, inspired by the story of another woman who successfully lost weight. Only this time it was not a "diet." She had learned about "dieting" with her prior weight loss attempts and knew that going on a diet meant eventually going off a diet. Marta made changes that she hoped would be permanent—reducing portion size, eliminating high fat foods, and not buying her weaknesses, cheese and pastries.

There are few long-term studies of commercial weight-loss programs. Despite the expense, many participants do not complete these programs, and most losers gain the weight back.

Marta also aimed to exercise for 45 minutes at least four times a week. Buying good walking shoes and having the level surface of a local track helped her avoid joint problems as she began her physical activity program.

Despite some setbacks, over the next 15 months, Marta gradually lost weight while her fitness improved. Now, Marta walks almost daily, covering four miles at a brisk pace. A year and a half after starting her program, she weighs 195 pounds, with a BMI of 28. Marta says that keeping the weight off requires constant attention to healthy eating and making sure that she gets regular exercise.

If you are naturally thin, you may have wondered how someone could spend money to lose weight, only to gain it all back again. If you are overweight, there is no mystery. You know how easy it is to gain weight, despite your efforts. Although it is a challenge to lose weight and keep it off, *it can be done.*

Researchers have interviewed successful weight losers, people who have lost many pounds and kept them off, trying to discover how they did it. What are their secrets? The findings are listed in Table 7.1. Importantly, almost all of them get regular exercise. Becoming physically active and losing weight can lower blood pressure, prevent Type 2 (adult-onset) diabetes, and reduce joint stress. Exercise not only helps you lose weight, it is essential for keeping it off.

The Wrong Metabolism for the Twenty-first Century

Scientists are just starting to unravel the biological mechanisms that regulate our body weight. Given how different our food intakes and activity patterns are day to day, our individual weights are amazingly constant. It appears we all have a certain weight that our body wants to be, called the *set point.* Your body regulates your weight around your set point, just as it adjusts your physiology to maintain your body temperature and the appropriate oxygen level in your bloodstream.

If you weigh less than your set point, your body craves food and slows your metabolism to conserve calories. And, when your weight is

---

TABLE 7.1   **Advice from Winners at Weight Loss**

Don't give up. Successful losers averaged five previous serious attempts at weight loss before success. They looked at their failed attempts as ways to learn things that contributed to their ultimate success.

Exercise moderately. Most exercised three or more times a week, and the majority walked.

No "diets." Changes in nutrition were gradual, and those changes fitted into their lifestyles. They ate at least three meals a day, plus snacks, choosing from low-fat, lower-calorie foods.

No gimmicks. Permanent weight loss did not come from pills, fat-blockers, fat-burners, prepackaged special diets, liquid supplements, or surgery.

Fifteen years ago, very low calorie diets were considered a popular and effective way to lose weight. What happened when the diet stopped? Three years after such a diet, researchers contacted almost 200 people who had lost an average of 50 pounds. Ninety percent had gained back most of their lost weight. *The strongest predictor of keeping the weight off was whether they exercised.*

The percentage of body fat is usually calculated using measured skinfold thickness, underwater weighing, or electrical impedance. Optimal for men is 14 to 18 percent, and for women it is 18 to 25 percent.

greater than your set point, you automatically eat less until your weight returns to your set point. Unfortunately, some of us have a set point that is too high for our own good health.

Studies with mice have identified specific genetic conditions that result in weight gain. For example, mice (and men) have a hormone, called leptin, that is made by fat cells and circulates in their (and our) bloodstreams. The leptin level is one of the ways body weight is regulated. When body fat and leptin levels are low, mice slow their metabolic rate and eat more. Conversely, when leptin and body fat levels are high, the mice eat less. Some mice have a hereditary lack of leptin, so their bodies react as though they had no body fat. Without any leptin, those mice get fatter and fatter. You can treat the mice by injecting them with the missing leptin. Then, like a normal mouse, they will stop gaining weight.

The discovery of leptin was an exciting breakthrough. Drug companies saw the potential of using leptin to treat obesity and paid more for its rights than the cost of a first-round draft choice. As you have probably guessed, humans are much more complicated than mice. Lack of leptin does not explain why we gain weight. So far, these research findings have not made it any easier to lose weight (unless you are a mouse). However, insight into obesity's physiology has given credence to weight gain being due to your metabolism and not lack of will power.

For many of us, our set point weight is higher than what is healthy. Remember our ancestors Cort and Corta from Chapter 1? Our bodies evolved when food was much more than 20 feet away in the refrigerator. Our ancient relatives were much more physically active, and their diets were lower in fat. They endured prolonged times when food was scarce. In those times, people with the higher set points were the lucky ones: they kept enough body fat to survive a famine. But times have changed, and high set points are out this millennium.

Today, a high set point means that you must work at not gaining an unhealthy amount of body fat. *Does this mean that losing weight is hopeless? No!* A well-known example is Oprah Winfrey. She lost weight using a very low calorie diet and showed off her new size six body on her talk show. However, she gained the weight back faster than you could say commercial break. Next time, she lost the weight gradually, a loss that she has maintained for years, using lifestyle changes: regular exercise and low-fat cooking. (And yes, a personal chef and her own exercise trainer do not hurt, either.)

Obesity in America

Obesity is a *big* problem for Americans and for people in most developed countries. You are considered obese when your weight is associated with significant health problems such as diabetes, high blood pressure, a high cholesterol level, and heart attacks. We used to determine normal weights by looking at height-and-weight charts. In the summer of 1998, the official definition of obesity was changed to be based on your body mass index, or BMI (Tables 7.2–7.4). With this new definition, more than half of U.S. adults are classified as obese, and that percentage grows each year.

How fat are we? In round figures, we're so fat that it makes us thick to our stomachs, we're breaking the pound barrier, and we live way beyond our seams—so that we go to great lengths to change our width.

The Costs of Obesity

Despite the many fat jokes, being overweight is not funny. It doubles the chance of heart disease, triples the risk of high blood pressure, and increases the likelihood of Type 2 (adult-onset) diabetes fivefold. Obesity even increases your risk for certain cancers. When the costs of obesity are weighed in, each additional pound of fat costs almost $200—a total for the nation of $100 billion a year.

TABLE 7.2   **Body Mass Index (BMI) and Obesity**

Obesity is when your weight harms your health, and it is based on the body mass index (BMI). Your BMI is calculated from your height and weight (see the example in Table 7.3), or you can find your weight category in Table 7.4. Using the BMI, we can directly compare people of different heights and frame sizes. Also, talking about your BMI can be less emotionally charged than discussing your weight or your percentage of body fat.

BMI	Weight Category
Less than 18.5	Underweight
18.5 to 24.9	Normal (healthiest weights)
25 to 29.9	Overweight (may harm health, especially with other risks for heart disease)
30 to 40	Obese (definite health risks)
More than 40	Extreme obesity (major health risks)

> ### TABLE 7.3   **Calculating Your Body Mass Index**
>
> Your BMI is your weight in kilograms divided by your height in meters squared. To calculate your value using pounds and inches, follow these steps:
> 1. Measure your height and weight: weight _____ pounds
>   height _____ inches
> 2. Multiply your weight (in pounds) by 703
> 3. Calculate (your height [in inches])^2
> 4. Divide the result in step 2 by the result in step 3, which gives you your BMI
>
> *For example:*
> 1. Marta weighed 247 pounds and stood 5 feet, 10 inches (or 70 inches) tall.
> 2. 247 lbs. × 703 = 173641
> 3. (70 inches)^2 = 4900
> 4. 173641 ÷ 4900 = 35.4 (her BMI)

How Weight Loss Happens

Weight loss happens when the number of calories you eat (what goes in) are fewer than the calories you burn (what goes out). You can look up the number of calories in foods, and for the other side of the equation, it helps to know about the three major ways your body uses calories (Figure 7.1).

TABLE 7.4   **BMI Categories for Different Heights and Weights**

	Optimal BMI = 22	Overweight BMI = 25	Obese BMI = 30	Extreme Obesity BMI = 40
4 ft 10 inches	105 lbs	120 lbs	144 lbs	191 lbs
5 ft 0 inches	112 lbs	128 lbs	153 lbs	205 lbs
5 ft 2 inches	120 lbs	137 lbs	164 lbs	219 lbs
5 ft 4 inches	128 lbs	146 lbs	175 lbs	233 lbs
5 ft 6 inches	136 lbs	155 lbs	186 lbs	248 lbs
5 ft 8 inches	144 lbs	164 lbs	197 lbs	263 lbs
5 ft 10 inches	153 lbs	174 lbs	209 lbs	279 lbs
6 ft 0 inches	162 lbs	185 lbs	222 lbs	295 lbs
6 ft 2 inches	171 lbs	195 lbs	233 lbs	311 lbs
6 ft 4 inches	180 lbs	206 lbs	247 lbs	329 lbs

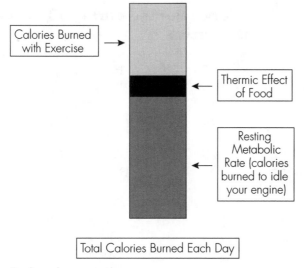

Figure 7.1 Daily caloric needs.

The largest number of calories goes to support your resting metabolic rate, or RMR. These calories are used to "idle your engine" and keep your organs and body tissues in working order. It is what you are burning right now, sitting still and reading this book. A much smaller number of calories is used to digest and absorb the nutrients you eat (which is called the thermic effect of food). You rev your metabolism each time you consume food. Even though the calories expended are few, you can take advantage of this effect by eating several small meals a day instead of one or two big ones.

For those of you with a BMI greater than 27, 7 out of 10 will have high blood pressure, diabetes, or abnormal blood fat levels.

The third way that you burn calories is by exercising. For the average person (and the above-average person like yourself), approximately 25 percent of the calories you burn in a day go to fuel physical activity. This is the part of the "calories out" equation over which we have the most control. The more active you are, the more calories you use. Regrettably for life in modern times, our bodies are fuel efficient. While that was good for your ancestors, it is bad for us. On foot, our bodies get 35 miles from each pound of body fat. (That would be more than 250 miles per gallon. Beat that, Detroit.) You do not have to work up a sweat to burn calories. When you run a mile, you burn about 100 calories, and you use almost the same number when you walk that distance. Walking just takes longer. Table 7.5 shows the number of calories burned with

TABLE 7.5	**Calories Burned during 30 Minutes of Exercise**		
Backpacking	250	Handball	330
Badminton	200	Hiking	180
Baseball	160	Horseback riding	200
Basketball	300	Mowing grass	140
Bicycling at 5.5 mph	150	Racquetball	300
Bicycling at 7 mph	200	Running at 5.5 mph	375
Bicycling at 12 mph	310	Running at 7 mph	500
Bowling	150	Sailing	150
Carpentry	135	Skiing	325
Chopping broccoli	100	Soccer	300
Chopping wood	250	Softball	150
Dancing	150	Swimming	180
Fencing	300	Tennis	270
Football	300	Volleyball	170
Gardening	150	Walking at 2 mph	120
Golfing (using cart)	120	Walking at 5 mph	270
Golfing (carrying clubs)	200		

different activities. Compare the number of calories you used in a half-hour walk (120–270 calories) with the calories in a piece of pie (300 calories) or cake (310 calories). Doesn't seem fair, does it?

Exercise also speeds up your metabolism for a few minutes after exertion (called the thermic effect of exercise). However, unless the exertion is prolonged (more than three hours) or extremely intense, the boost in metabolism lasts just 30 minutes and amounts to an extra 10 to 25 calories. The only way that regular exercise can boost your metabolic rate for a longer time is if you build more muscle.

You do not have to lose all your extra body fat to see health benefits. Often, just losing 10 percent of your total weight will improve your health.

Activities That Help You Lose Weight

Barbara is a 64-year-old woman in good general health. She came to the clinic for an annual exam. Barbara looks younger than her age, and she takes pride in her appearance. She has gained several pounds over the last few years despite cutting back on what she eats. Though she feels well, she said that she would like to lose some weight.

Barbara's blood pressure was up slightly from a year ago at 157/88 mm Hg (normal is below 140/90 mm Hg). Her height was 5 feet, 5 inches, and she weighed 165 pounds. Her body mass index was 27.5. Measuring her skin folds showed that she had 34 percent body fat (165 pounds = 109 pounds of lean, or nonfat, tissue + 56 pounds of body fat, giving a percent body fat of 56 ÷ 165 = 34 percent). The remainder of her physical examination was normal.

The only modest abnormality in her laboratory results was a blood sugar level of 120 mg/dL (normal is less than 110 mg/dL). Barbara recalled that her mother developed diabetes late in life, and because diabetes runs in families, Barbara is at greater risk. Her slightly increased blood sugar level also means that she may be headed for diabetes, a course she can change by exercising and losing body fat.

One of the reasons that our weight goes up along with our age is that we gradually lose muscle. Our resting metabolic rate (the number of calories burned at rest) depends largely on the amount of muscle we have. The sizes of our internal organs are all pretty similar: what does differ is the amount of muscle in our bodies. The more muscle, the higher the resting metabolic rate. In general, men have higher metabolic rates than women. That difference is all due to men having more muscle than women.

As we age, we lose muscle fibers, and muscles get smaller—unless we exercise regularly. If we stay active, we will not lose (and can even build) muscle. That way, our metabolism will not decrease as we get older. You also lose muscle when you are losing body weight—again, unless you exercise. If you are physically active while losing weight, you will preserve your muscles, and the weight you lose will be mostly body fat.

Barbara had never been a regular exerciser. Initially, she purchased several videotape workouts because she thought that she would feel less embarrassed exercising at home. However, she found herself too distracted by what needed to be done around the house. After several weeks, she moved to plan B and joined a local gym. There, her workouts seemed to go much faster. After some initial instruction on strength training, she added it to her workouts. Barbara's strength increased in just a few weeks. Although her weight did not change, she lost one dress size and felt much better.

There are advantages and disadvantages for each type of physical activity. Theoretically, to lose weight, the best exercise program would be a combination of aerobic exercise to burn calories and increase endurance, plus weight training to add strength, build muscle, and increase your resting metabolic rate.

Adult-onset or Type 2, diabetes is the most common type of diabetes. It runs in families and is also associated with being overweight.

Which home exercise equipment burns the most calories? It depends. Most of us can use a stationary cycle or walk on a treadmill. Other equipment requires you to learn how to use it, and not everybody can get the knack of things. For example, we found that some experienced runners found it difficult to use a cross-country ski machine. So, for them, using a treadmill burned more calories. Treadmill exercise and cross-country ski machines burn the most calories (at the same training heart rate), followed by then a stationary cycle, and then a rowing machine. While these findings might be interesting, you should select your home exercise equipment based on what you enjoy doing, rather than on any theoretical calorie-burning advantage.

Obesity is when your body mass index is 30 or more, which usually means more than 30 pounds over a healthy weight.

Training guidelines for beginning aerobic or endurance activities (such as brisk walking, jogging, aerobics, cycling, or swimming) are shown in Table 7.6. Typically, these activities burn more calories per minute than lifting weights. However, they do not build much muscle, so endurance activities will not change your resting metabolic rate.

The recommendations in Table 7.6 are the same whether your BMI is 18 or 40. If you are overweight, usually it will take less exercise for you to achieve your training level—just as if a normal-weight person were wearing a heavy backpack. Do not let that discourage you. Whatever your fitness level, it can only improve, and you are burning a few more calories by carrying that backpack.

Weight lifting to build strength and muscle raises the number of calories that your body burns each day. Pumping iron also has the advantage of causing changes more quickly than does endurance training. When you start a weight-lifting program, you become stronger in a couple of weeks, long before your endurance improves from aerobic conditioning. Seeing your strength increase early on can help you stay with the program.

The truth is, while a combination of aerobic exercise and strength training may be ideal, it is no good unless you do it. Almost any kind of exercise burns calories and improves your health. For most of us, it is

---

TABLE 7.6   **Guidelines for Aerobic or Endurance Conditioning**

Workout intensity:
- At a 3 to 5 (moderate or somewhat strong) on a scale of 1 (very light exercise) to 10 (exercising as hard as you can)
- So you have enough breath to talk easily (you may not have enough to sing, though)
- At a heart rate approximately 70 percent of your maximal heart rate (your maximal heart rate = 220 − your age)

Workout frequency should be at least three times a week for a minimum of 30 minutes each time. For fat loss, daily exercise is best.

It takes months to get in shape, and training more intensely will not speed the process. Your endurance will increase slowly over about four months, but add an additional month for every year that you have been inactive.

As your aerobic endurance increases, it will take more work to reach your training intensity, but the intensity indicators listed above will stay the same.

most important to find an activity we enjoy and can fit into our daily routine.

When seen a few months later, Barbara's body weight was down three pounds. Although she had not consciously tried to cut calories, Barbara found that she had eliminated many high-fat items. When we checked her skin folds, her total body fat was eight pounds less, and she had gained five pounds of muscle. Her BMI was 27, and her percentage of body fat had gone from 34 to 30 percent (48 ÷ 162 = 30 percent). Her fasting blood sugar was normal. Although her body was not "hard," it was definitely firmer. She said that her new-found strength was accompanied by a greater feeling of self-confidence. Her spirits were lifted along with the weights.

For women, strength training, more than aerobic exercise, increases self-confidence and self-esteem.

Apple and Pear Shapes

Bill is a commercial real estate sales associate, and he just turned 40. Although it was one of those dreaded birthdays that ends in a zero, he always considered himself healthy. It was a real shock when one of his coworkers, who was only a few years older, died suddenly from a heart attack. Bill came in for a physical examination at the insistence of his wife, who half-jokingly said that he should either see a doctor or double his life insurance coverage.

Bill's weight had slowly increased since college, especially over the last four years. Office work and family life ate up his time, while he was eating up a meat and potatoes diet, high in saturated fats. Lately, Bill was buying jeans with the relaxed fit and had developed what his wife called his "little beer belly."

At 6 feet and 1 inch tall, Bill weighed 230 pounds, giving him a body mass index of 30. His physical examination, other than his amount and distribution of body fat, was normal. His wife was right about the weight around his midsection. His waist size was two inches larger than the distance around his hips.

Some men and women have what is called abdominal obesity. Figure 7.2 shows the two main types of obesity: apple-shaped, or abdominal, obesity, and pear-shaped, or lower body, obesity. Those with abdominal

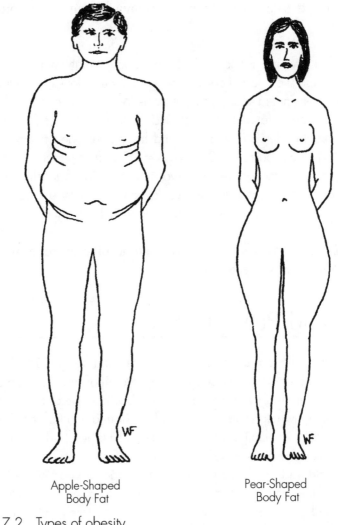

Apple-Shaped
Body Fat

Pear-Shaped
Body Fat

Figure 7.2   Types of obesity.

obesity have more fat in their midsection, both in their abdominal wall and around their internal organs. Observing the front and side view will often tell you where your extra fat is stored. You can know for sure by comparing your waist and hip size. If your waist measurement divided by your hip measurement is more than 0.95 for men and 0.8 for women, then you have abdominal obesity.

Abdominal fat stores are especially unhealthy and increase your risk for heart disease, high blood pressure, and diabetes. Because abdominal obesity is so risky, a waist measurement of more than 40 inches for men and 35 inches for women is considered obese, even if your BMI is less than 30. Although abdominal fat cells are more risky, they are also easier to lose. In general, if you are overweight and start exercising (without cutting back on calories), you will not lose much weight—maybe a couple of pounds. Abdominal obesity is the exception to that rule. Abdominal fat deposits are often reduced with a consistent program of walking, cycling, jogging, or swimming. It is as if those abdominal fat cells are more active—both in causing health problems and in shrinking with regular exercise.

We discussed Bill's findings and that regular aerobic exercise, even without dieting, would increase his fitness, burn calories, and probably decrease his risky abdominal fat. At age 40, with only an elevated cholesterol level as a risk factor for coronary heart disease, Bill did not need an exercise stress test before beginning a vigorous exercise program. However, he had been an athlete in high school and was trained in the old-school exercise philosophy of "no pain, no gain." So, he did need information about how hard to exercise and what to expect as he got in shape (Table 7.6).

Bill began a program of brisk walking four times a week, with additional upper- and lower-body strength training. He and his wife began to exercise together, and they arrived at a schedule in which they walked for 40 minutes most mornings and went to a health club one weekday and on weekends. During the following year, Bill's weight slowly decreased. He found himself eating healthier foods. After working out, it seemed easier to resist a midmorning Danish, and the lunchtime roast beef sandwiches did not look as good to him as they had before. He did not miss his few weekend beers, and their 150 calories per can. Fourteen months after he was first seen, Bill weighed 30 pounds less, his BMI was 26, and his cholesterol levels also were improved.

To lose a pound of body fat, you must burn an extra 3,500 calories.

The Truth about Miracle Diets

Bookstores have rows and rows of diet books. In an hour of channel surfing, you can see infomercials about fat-busting chemicals, the latest weight-loss plans, and what is new in calorie-burning exercise equipment. Each describes the newest "breakthrough" for weight loss, complete with testimonials and before and after pictures. The facts are that almost any diet will result in weight loss . . . at least for a while.

Do not be misled when you lose six or seven pounds the first week of your latest diet. There is a reason for that rapid weight loss—and it is not a miracle diet. Your body has two types of fuel stores: *sugars*, stored with water in the form of glycogen in your muscles and liver, and *fat* (and you know where that is stored). When you first cut back on calories, your body uses the stored sugars. As those water-packed sugars are burned, water is lost in your urine. It is that water loss that accounts for your initial rapid weight loss. Although you lost weight the first week, you did not lose much body fat. If you increase your calorie intake, your body will remake the sugars, and you will regain the lost water weight.

Usually, by the second or third week of a diet, your weight loss slows down. At that point you may be getting tired of your miracle diet. As you revert to your prior eating habits, your lost weight also comes back. You are at your original weight just in time for the next break-through diet that hits the best-seller list.

What It Takes for Weight Loss

Most of us will lose weight while eating 1,000 to 1,200 calories a day (for women) or 1,200 to 1,500 calories a day (for men). Those calories should be portioned into three meals a day, plus snacks. (Calories eaten standing up do count.) Keep your food choices low in fat and aim for less than 30 percent of your total calories coming from fat.

For most of us, long-term weight loss means regular exercise, eating a low-fat diet, and changing some of our eating habits. To lose weight, try to eat approximately 500 calories less than the number of calories you need each day. For women, you can lose weight eating 1,000 to 1,200 calories each day, and that number is 1,200 to 1,500 calories for men. More is not better, when it comes to decreasing your calories. Cutting back more than 500 calories each day can make it *harder* to lose weight. If you reduce your calorie intake too much, your body will think it is starving and slow your metabolic rate. Changing a lifetime of unhealthy eating habits is difficult. Try the suggestions in Table 7.7, or consider a weight-loss program (Table 7.8). Regular daily exercise plus moderate calorie restriction will result in a gradual loss of one to two pounds of body fat each week.

Advice for Very Overweight Individuals

The more body fat you have, the greater the risk to your health. When you are 100 or more pounds overweight (or your BMI is more than 40),

---

TABLE 7.7 **Healthy Eating Habits**

Eat three meals a day. Going many hours without eating trains your body to store fat.

Do not deprive yourself. If you are craving a certain food, it is okay to indulge. Just cut back on other calories or exercise more.

Keep records of what you eat. It can be surprising to total up your calories and see how many are in a croissant or a slice of cheese.

Slow your eating and pay attention to portion size. What we eat is often guided by habit, not hunger.

Look at food labels for total calories and the percentage of calories from fat. "Low fat" does not always mean "low calorie." Keeping fat intake at less than 30 percent of total calories is important, but so is the total number of calories.

Think about whether you would be helped by a weight loss program. Changing eating habits is difficult. A little help may be just what you need.

Do not forget to exercise. Exercise burns calories and prevents muscle loss. The benefits of physical activity reinforce your healthy eating habits.

---

you are a likely candidate for high blood pressure, diabetes, degenerative arthritis, breathing problems, and heart disease. If this describes you, then you should see your health care provider before beginning an exercise and weight loss program.

When you are given the go ahead for physical activity, you have a few additional considerations. Because of your weight, you are more likely to have a joint injury when exercising, and your movements may be restricted. For those reasons, swimming or stationary cycling are often good exercise choices because they put less stress on your back, hips, knees, ankles, and feet. Also, a gradual walking program, using supportive shoes and a level surface, aimed at achieving a two-mile distance each workout, can be effective. Some very overweight people are uncomfortable about appearing in bathing suits, and many pools have specific swim times for people who are obese. The references at the end of this book have other resources to help.

Finally, because you are well insulated, you are more likely to overheat when exercising. Drink enough fluids before working out to make your urine light yellow or clear, and while you are exercising, have an additional eight ounces of liquid every 30 minutes.

	TABLE 7.8 **Programs for Weight Loss**			
Program	**Program Content**	**Frequency of Meetings**	**Provider Qualifications**	**Approximate Cost**
One-on-One Counseling				
Dietitians	Individualized diet plan and counseling about nutrition, eating habits, and physical activity	Contact frequency based on your needs and goals; usually begins at once per week	Registered dietitians	Varies; inquire with each health care provider
Personal trainers	Nutrition plan and supervised exercise at a fitness facility	Contact frequency based on your needs and goals; usually begins at once per week	Training and certification varies	Varies; need to inquire
Self-help				
Overeaters Anonymous	Nonprofit 12-step support group; specific weight loss plans usually not provided	Weekly meetings	Members conduct activities	None (donations welcomed)
TOPS (Take Off Pounds Sensibly)	Uses food exchange lists for its nutrition program	Weekly meetings	Volunteer chapter leaders	Approximately $16/week
Commercial Weight Loss				
Jenny Craig, Inc.	Individual counseling supplemented with audio and videotapes; sells own proprietary food line	Twice per week	Employees have more than 40 hours of training by the company and receive ongoing support	Varies with duration of enrollment and amount of weight loss; average cost approximately $300
Weight Watchers International, Inc.	Weekly classes that provide support and advice on nutrition, exercise, and behavior change; uses an exercise guidance handbook; supplemental newspaper, books, and magazines available	One hour per week	Group leaders are company-trained "gradu-ates" who must maintain their own weight loss	Initial registration fee and weekly attendance fee

TABLE 7.8 **Programs for Weight Loss** (continued)				
Program	**Program Content**	**Frequency of Meetings**	**Provider Qualifications**	**Approximate Cost**
Community Based				
Hospital-, church-, or community-center-based programs	Advice about nutrition, behavior change, and physical activity	Weekly for a specified number of sessions	Usually dietitian(s) or health educators	Varies

What about Diet Drugs?

Eventually, there may be a place for drug treatment of obesity. It would be great if we could "fix" it with a pill—just as we give medications for high blood pressure and high cholesterol levels. But right now, there are two big problems with using drugs. First, for most people, keeping the weight off would mean staying on the drug for life. When dexfenfluramine (Redux) and Fen-Phen (fenteramine and phenteramine) were prescribed, many people lost weight. Those drugs were found to have significant side effects and have been taken off the market. Once the drugs were stopped, almost all who lost weight gained it back. Having that happen is not unexpected. You would expect your blood pressure to go up if you discontinued treatment, and your blood sugar would increase if you stopped drug therapy of diabetes. So, why should your weight not go back up when you stop diet drugs? Currently, no drugs are approved for long-term treatment of obesity.

When it comes to body weight, society confuses looking good with being healthy. Look at ancient Greek statues. Those women would be wearing size 12 or 14, not the size 2 of fashion models.

Second, all weight-loss drugs have potential side effects that can be severe and much worse than being overweight. If we had an effective weight-loss drug, it might be prescribed for millions of people, many more than take any other type of prescription medication (remember, half the population is obese). With so many people getting the drug, we are sure to see the side effects, even if they are rare.

Weight-loss drugs should not ever be used by those who want to lose a few pounds to "look better."

The story of dexfenfluramine (Redux) illustrates the risks and shows that if something seems too good to be true, it probably is. In 1996, Redux was approved as a weight-loss drug by the U.S. Food and

Orlistat is a new weight-loss drug that reduces your ability to digest and absorb fats from your diet. Its side effects are gas and diarrhea—similar to what is caused by the nonabsorbable fat, castor oil.

Drug Administration. It was the first new weight-loss medication in 25 years. Redux appeared on the cover of *Time* magazine and was hailed as a miracle drug. However, because it was prescribed so widely, rare side effects that were not observed during the drug company's initial tests were seen. Less than a year after its release, it was withdrawn from the market because it sometimes caused life-threatening types of heart disease.

Most people with too much body fat have a metabolic problem and not a lack of will power. Those of us who gain weight easily need even more will power to resist the temptations of modern-day rich, fattening foods and sedentary lifestyles. To be at our healthiest weight, we need to eat low-fat foods, pay attention to our eating habits and total calories, and get regular exercise.

Bottom Lines

The lifestyle changes that lead to weight loss—eating a balanced, low-fat diet and exercising regularly—improve your health in many ways, in addition to helping you lose weight. Exercise burns calories and preserves your muscle mass, so the weight lost is primarily body fat. Those with the additional health risks of abdominal, or apple-shaped, obesity may particularly benefit from regular exercise. While a single bout of physical activity has little effect on the calories you burn when not exercising, strength or weight training can build muscle tissue and in doing so increase your resting metabolic rate. We doubt that any weight loss medication will ever be able to do as much for weight loss as regular exercise.

Chapter 8

Exercise to Lower Blood Pressure

As the cuff around his arm deflated, the reading on the screen flashed 168/96 mm Hg. J. Michael, a 47-year-old, self-proclaimed "high-powered" attorney, discovered his blood pressure was high when he checked it at the local drug store. He hadn't seen a physician in a long time and decided it was time to get some professional help.

He talked to clients and friends for a few days, trying to locate the "best" physician. Then he came across an announcement in the newspaper requesting volunteers with hypertension to enroll in a study designed to treat high blood pressure with exercise. The requirements were to have elevated blood pressure and not to have exercised regularly (not more than once per week) during the past six months. No problem. J. Michael's main activities were wrestling with legal documents and an occasional courtroom brawl. He couldn't remember when he last exerted himself physically. He had not even mowed the lawn since he hired a lawn maintenance service when his son was born three years before.

J. Michael's dietary habits were in need of a major overhaul. He often skipped breakfast. During the day he ate on the run, subsisting on fast food hamburgers and large servings of vegetables—in the form of french fries. From the fruit food group, he chose ketchup, the kind in the single-serving, user-friendly plastic packages, which he generously splattered over his burger and fries. After work, he downed a few scotch and sodas to help him relax. On the weekends he had wine before, during, and after dinner. He justified this by believing alcohol helped him unwind after a rigorous week of behind-the-desk work. Seeing his high blood pressure reading on the pharmacy's machine left him feeling quite vulnerable. Hoping to be around to watch his young son (and future law partner) grow up, he called the university and applied to enter the research study.

When not counseling and interviewing employees and job applicants for the state, Sarah, a 37-year-old single mother, was busy shuttling her 9-year-old son and 11-year-old daughter to various sporting events and after-school activities—soccer in the fall, basketball in the winter, and baseball and softball in the spring, not to mention various youth group meetings. In the summer, there were sport camps, theater workshops, and the mall.

Sarah's children were very active. Sarah was not. Her main exercise was driving, driving, and more driving. She enjoyed going to the movies and having dinner with friends, but this was when she had a free evening, and there weren't many of those. Her last regular physical activity was during a college physical education class. Sarah had smoked one-half pack of cigarettes each day since high school, "but never around the children." Her eating habits were like her children's diets. In fact she often finished their food while on the road during shuttle trips.

Sarah's weight had increased about 20 pounds over the past five years. During a routine dental appointment, Sarah's dentist measured her blood pressure and found it to be 150/100 mm Hg. She was referred for a medical evaluation and treatment.

J. Michael and Sarah were diagnosed with the same problem, hypertension. But before we discuss their problems any further, you need to know what hypertension really is.

What Is Hypertension?

Systolic Pressure

Diastolic Pressure

Hypertension has little to do with feeling 'hyper' and not much to do with being 'tense'. Hypertension is another term for high blood pressure and usually has no symptoms. But how high is high? Today, hypertension is diagnosed when the top number (the systolic blood pressure) is consistently at or above 140 millimeters of mercury (mm Hg) and/or the lower number (the diastolic pressure) is at or above 90 mm Hg. Because everyone's blood pressure changes over the course of a day, before your blood pressure is considered high, it should be taken at least three times, several days to weeks apart, and only after you have rested

TABLE 8.1	**Categories of Blood Pressure Levels (in mm Hg)**	
Blood Pressure (mm Hg)	**The Blood Pressure Category**	**What to Do?**
Below 120/80	Optimal—the best	Recheck in one to two years
Below 130/85	Normal	Recheck in one year
130–139/85–89	High-normal range	Lower your risk factors, recheck in six months
140–159/90–99	Mild hypertension	Danger! Confirm with three checks, then treat and recheck
160–179/100–109	Moderate hypertension	Get help now!
180+/110+	Severe hypertension	Immediate and major help needed, often with more than one medication

in a seated position for at least five minutes. Table 8.1 lists categories of different blood pressure levels.

A level of 140/90 mm Hg indicates mild hypertension, and it triggers a physician's awareness of the problem. Medical evaluation is necessary, and if your blood pressure remains at or above this level, treatment is needed. When blood pressures reaches the moderate to severe range, treatment should begin immediately. However, if you have heart disease or when other risks for heart and blood vessel disease are present, such as diabetes, blood pressure may be treated at the high normal range (130/85 mm Hg).

High blood pressure affects approximately 50 million Americans. That means more than one out of five adults in the United States has hypertension. Since high blood pressure usually causes no symptoms, it silently damages our blood vessels and organs, until severe injury has accumulated. This leads to heart attacks, heart failure (the heart becomes a less efficient pump), stroke (a brain attack), blood vessel narrowing, and kidney failure. The higher your blood pressure, the quicker and greater the harm it can cause.

Also, high blood pressure intensifies the damage done to the body by other problems such as a high cholesterol level, cigarette smoking, and diabetes. Although drugs can effectively reduce blood pressure, nearly three-fourths of Americans who have hypertension are either not treated or not treated well enough.

Systolic and Diastolic Pressure

Blood is always being pumped by your heart through your arteries. You can think of this blood flow as a river with waves that pulsate with each heartbeat. Blood pressure simply measures the force of these waves. The systolic pressure (upper number) measures the top of the wave, and the diastolic pressure (lower number) gauges the bottom. To complicate matters, since this river of blood is contained in a flexible pipe (your arteries), the systolic pressure is also related to the flexibility of your blood vessels. So, the harder your heart pumps or the stiffer your arteries are, the higher your systolic pressure will be.

On the other hand, diastolic blood pressure occurs as the heart relaxes (right before and after it beats). But because your arteries have muscles around their walls, the artery diameter can change. This is important because the ability to change the size of the arteries allows you to direct blood flow to vital organs during rest, or increase blood flow to muscles during physical exertion. If all our arteries were in the relaxed state, the vessels would be too large for the blood supply, blood pressure would plummet, and we would faint, or even worse, die of lack of blood flow to the brain and heart. When blood vessels dilate too much or you have too little blood volume to "fit" in your blood vessels, you have what is referred to as cardiovascular shock. The diastolic pressure is the measure of the amount of constriction or relaxation of your arteries. Diastolic hypertension causes a strain on your heart by forcing it to work harder to deliver blood to the body's vital organs and tissues.

What Causes High Blood Pressure?

Blood pressure naturally rises when you exercise, drink a few cups of regular coffee, or sit in the car as your 15-year-old takes the wheel for the first time. However, these relatively brief blood pressure elevations are not harmful to most people. It is only when the systolic and/or diastolic blood pressure remain elevated at rest that there is risk of damage. This continual elevation leads directly to heart attacks, strokes, narrowing of blood vessels, and problems with vision.

For only a small minority of those with hypertension does high blood pressure have a cause. It can result from the body's excessive production of hormones (such as thyroid hormone and adrenal gland hormones) or from problems with the kidney's blood supply or the kidney itself. In addition, use of certain drugs, including birth control pills, over-the-counter decongestants, and even nonsteroidal anti-inflammatory medications such as ibuprofen, can raise blood pressure. However, for 95 percent of those with hypertension, the cause is unknown.

Now, when doctors can't identify a specific reason to have high blood pressure, it has to be called something. You can't just say this person has high blood pressure. It needs a name. So 95 percent of the people with high blood pressure have what is referred to as *essential hypertension*. What this really means is that we have "essentially" no idea why most patients have high blood pressure. But there are a few clues. We do know that elevated blood pressure is rarely found in less-industrialized nations, and researchers have noticed that certain lifestyle factors appear responsible for the high rate of hypertension in the United States.

Lifestyle Factors and Hypertension

Less modern societies than ours have vastly different diets than we do. Unlike our cave relatives, Cort and Corta, we serve up many processed and fast food items, which are typically loaded with salt and fat. Also, most of us in industrialized countries have jobs that cannot be defined as *work* . . . . you know, the kinds of jobs that people had before the industrial revolution. These jobs required people to expend energy by using their muscles, which challenged their cardiovascular system. Over the past 60 years, many more people began to earn a salary while sitting at a desk, standing behind a counter, checking inventory, and driving equipment. While at home there are countless labor-saving devices. Entertainment is often achieved by pushing the buttons on a TV remote control. For these reasons, high blood pressure has become a big problem in the United States. Table 8.2 lists some of the lifestyle factors that can raise blood pressure.

```
┌─────────────────────────────────────────────┐
│  TABLE 8.2  Hypertension Risk Factors:       │
│             "The Usual Suspects"             │
│                                               │
│  • Drinking excessive amounts of alcohol     │
│  • Eating too much salt                      │
│  • Having too much body fat                  │
│  • Smoking tobacco                           │
│  • Exercising too little                     │
└─────────────────────────────────────────────┘
```

Suspect #1: Alcohol

Research has shown that moderate alcohol intake actually has some cardiovascular benefits. But just because a small amount is good, more is not better! In fact, if we measure the potential benefits of alcohol use against its harmful effects, there is no contest. Alcohol is a big loser! Despite the benefits of a small amount of red wine or similar amount of spirits each day, millions of hospitalizations are alcohol related. Excessive alcohol intake is a risk for developing hypertension and can block the beneficial effects of exercise and blood pressure medication. Alcohol is the number one drug problem among our youth, and problem drinking, drinking and driving, and chronic illness due to alcohol use take a terrible toll on the drinker, his or her family, and society.

If you enjoy alcohol, limit your daily intake to an equivalent of 1 ounce (most men) or $^{1}/_{2}$ ounce (women and smaller men). An ounce of alcohol is the same as drinking 2 ounces of 100 proof whiskey, two 5 ounce glasses of wine, or two 12 ounce bottles of beer. More alcohol than this will increase your risk of developing high blood pressure.

Suspect #2: Salt

Salt is a combination of sodium (Na) and chloride (Cl), and all of us need it to survive. The sodium portion helps us retain fluid in our blood, muscle, and other tissues. However, the problem is that much of the food we eat, especially processed foods, contain way too much salt. The human body is already loaded with sodium, and our hormones regulate and conserve the salt, even when it is scarce.

The risks of eating a high-salt diet still are hotly debated, and a few scientists think a high-sodium diet is no big deal. For some people, this is true. However, there is a significant group of people with high blood pressure who are salt sensitive. For them, it is a very big deal. If you are salt sensitive, a high-sodium diet results in high blood pressure.

The average American eats approximately 10 grams of salt each day, most (75 percent) of which comes from eating processed foods. This is a lot more than we need. Studies have linked heart, kidney, and blood vessel damage among those with hypertension to their high intake of dietary salt. In fact, just reducing your sodium intake can lower blood pressure. However, a word of caution. If you try to stay on a no-salt diet, you will be limited to eating something like white rice and apples. Fortunately, it is not necessary to severely restrict sodium from your diet, and because of food processing, it is nearly impossible.

For all of us, it is important to always taste the food before reaching for the salt shaker. Experiment with herbs and spices to add flavor. If you already have high blood pressure or want to prevent hypertension, don't even use salt. Cut out salty convenience foods such as chips, canned soups, and processed meats. Lastly, by reducing the salt in recipes by one-half, you can greatly lower your daily salt intake to about 6,000 milligrams (6 grams). That is similar to taking in about 2,400 mg of sodium (check out the food label) or about 1 teaspoon of salt per day.

Suspect #3: Fat

A diet that is high in saturated fat can raise your blood pressure. Likewise a diet that is rich in fruits, vegetables, and low in saturated and total fat can help treat and prevent high blood pressure from ever occurring. If you are overweight, losing 10 pounds can significantly reduce your risk of developing high blood pressure.

One way to determine your hypertension risk is to calculate your body mass index (BMI). To do this, take your body weight in kilograms (1 pound = .45 kilograms) and divide it by your height in meters squared (1 inch = .026 meters). When your BMI reaches 27 or higher, your risk of developing high blood pressure increases. Table 7.3 in Chapter 7 shows you how to calculate your BMI. If you don't want to flip through the pages or do the math, check your waist size. When your waist reaches or exceeds 40 inches (for men) or 35 inches (for women), you increase your chance of developing hypertension.

Suspect #4: Smoking

Add "raising blood pressure" to the long list of harmful effects of smoking cigarettes and using chewing tobacco. Blood pressure will rise after smoking just one cigarette! When you use tobacco products, all your hard work and use of medication to bring down your blood pressure will literally go up in smoke!

Exercise and Hypertension

The more active and the more fit you are, the lower your blood pressure will be. This remarkable association is even true for children as young as 5 and 6 years old. When researchers observed the endurance of preadolescent and adolescent children on a treadmill and measured their blood pressure, the fittest groups of boys and girls had the lowest blood pressure. Also, adults of all ages who are more fit and maintain their fitness are about half as likely as unfit adults to develop high blood pressure in the future.

Unfortunately, about 80 percent of the people in the United States fail to get enough exercise. This includes children, who are becoming increasingly less fit. Today, many grade schools actually limit the availability and time for physical education classes. If we could improve the physical fitness of our children, millions of future adults might not have high blood pressure.

Does Blood Pressure Treatment Help Prevent Disease?

Lowering high blood pressure saves lives and prevents the complications of hypertension. About 30 years ago, it was shown that treatment of high blood pressure resulted in a 75 percent lowering of stroke and heart failure rates. Since that time many other studies have shown that treatment has similar benefits, resulting in a longer life span with less illness.

What is truly important about treatment is that you do not need to have a large reduction in blood pressure to gain significant benefit. Although you want your blood pressure to be in the normal or optimal range, even small reductions—about 5 mm Hg—can reduce the risk of organ damage. But the greatest reductions in risk are when your blood pressure is below 140/90 mm Hg.

Medication for Treating Hypertension

Blood pressure medications are effective, and as physicians we write prescriptions for these drugs nearly every day. There are different types (or classes) of these drugs, and each class lowers blood pressure in a somewhat different way. For example, many work by dilating arteries. Some reduce the amount of water in our bloodstream, while others block the effect of blood pressure–raising hormones.

But the downside of all drug treatment is the side effects. All of these drugs can cause dizziness or a feeling of lightheadedness. Beyond this, each class of drugs can have unique side effects (Table 8.3). While hypertension usually has no symptoms, blood pressure medications often do. In fact, side effects are one reason why many people (about 50 percent) do not take their blood pressure medicine as prescribed. In addition to all this, blood pressure medications cost money. Some brands cost a lot! The cost of using just one of the newer blood pressure medications

TABLE 8.3 **Drugs to Lower Blood Pressure**

Drug Class	Generic Examples	Potential Side Effects
Diuretics	Hydrochlorothiazide, furosemide	Dizziness, muscle cramps, low potassium levels
Beta blockers	Propranolol, atenolol, metoprolol	Fatigue, impotence, reduced exercise capacity
Alpha-beta blocker	Labetalol	Dizziness, weakness, fatigue
Central alpha agonists	Clonidine, guanfacine, guanabenz	Fatigue, confusion, sleepiness
Vasodilators	Hydralazine, minoxidil	Headache, fluid retention, rapid heart rate
Calcium channel blockers	Verapamil, diltiazem, nifedipine, felodipine, amlodipine	Constipation, fluid retention and leg swelling, headache, flushing
ACE inhibitors	Captopril, enalapril, lisinopril, ramipril	Cough, abnormal taste, headache
Angiotensin II blockers	Valsartan, losartan, telmisartan	Headache (probably lowest rate of side effects of any drug class)
Alpha blockers	Doxazosin, prazosin	Headache, dizziness

can be nearly $1,000 each year. Table 8.3 lists typical blood pressure medication classes and some generic names and common side effects.

Recommended Medication

Your health care provider is in the best position to answer your questions about which medication is best for you, because we are all unique and have different needs. Some drugs cause more unwanted side effects if you have an underlying medical condition. Other medications are chosen because they not only lower blood pressure, but can treat another problem such as migraine headaches or a heart rhythm disturbance.

The two drugs recommended most often by experts as first-line treatment for hypertension are diuretics and beta blockers. Diuretics, commonly referred to as water pills, lower your blood pressure by eliminating sodium and water via the urine. But diuretics can cause dizziness when too much water is removed, and they can reduce your body's level of potassium, which can lead to muscle cramps and heart rhythm disturbances. Because of this, high-potassium foods and/or potassium-containing pills or solutions often are prescribed when diuretics are used. Also, using diuretics means you will be a more frequent visitor to the bathroom. This will occur during the day . . . and night . . . and night again. And, in high doses, diuretics can worsen certain risk factors for heart disease by increasing your cholesterol level and making your blood sugar level more difficult to control.

Beta blockers work by counteracting the effect of adrenaline. Adrenaline and related hormones (epinephrine and norepinephrine) are constantly circulating through our bodies and are contained in certain nerve endings, where they serve as nerve impulse transmitters. These hormones stimulate the heart to beat faster and harder and cause some of our blood vessels to become narrower. The effects are due to the hormone attaching to specialized submicroscopic structures called beta receptors. Adrenaline fits into the beta receptor like a key fitting into a lock. When adrenaline slides into the receptor, the heart rate quickens and certain arteries clamp down. Beta blockers counteract the adrenaline in our body by competing with these adrenaline keys for the lock of the beta receptor, thus blocking the action of the hormones. So, when beta blockers are used, heart rates slow and blood pressure drops. The higher the dose, the greater the effect.

Now, beta blockers are wonderful drugs. They are known to reduce heart attack rates and lengthen life span for those with heart disease. Unfortunately a high proportion of people report side effects such as fatigue, reduced physical endurance, nightmares, depression, and impotence (Table 8.3). Furthermore, beta blockers can worsen asthma, elevate blood sugar levels among those with diabetes, and result in abnormal cholesterol levels. And they are among the best drugs! Although some newer medications have fewer side effects, they are much more expensive.

J. Michael entered the blood pressure study. He was placed on a calcium channel blocker to lower his blood pressure and began a physical activity program under the watchful eye of the exercise physiologist. He rode a stationary exercycle for 35 minutes, three times each week, for 12 weeks. He warmed up for 5 of those minutes, pedaled the exercycle at a perceived exertion of 3 (on a scale of 0 to 10) for 25 minutes, and cooled down by riding at a very low level for an additional 5 minutes. After 12 weeks, he lost six pounds of fat, gained two pounds of muscle, and his fitness improved. From 168/96 mm Hg, J. Michael's blood pressure dropped to 124/84 mm Hg. And he was able to discontinue the medication without any problems with blood pressure control.

During an examination two years later, he reported changing his eating habits. He now eats a low-fat breakfast, avoids fast food restaurants, and selects several portions of fruits and vegetables each day. His use of alcohol has declined to a beer with dinner once or twice each week. He occasionally falls off the "exercise wagon," and when he does, his blood pressure climbs into the hypertensive range (he monitors his blood pressure at home). Currently, he is exercising five times each week, does not take medication, and has a second child to enjoy.

To sum it up, J. Michael had three major risks that led to his hypertension: (1) too much alcohol, (2) a poor diet that contained excessive amounts of salt and fat and too few vegetables and fruits (foods that help reduce blood pressure), and (3) no physical activity. He was able to change his drinking habits with encouragement from his wife and physician. Knowing that he has a problem with "choices" at fast food restaurants when he is hungry ("I'll eat almost anything when I'm hungry"), J. Michael vowed to avoid these eating establishments altogether. Two years after completing the study, he grades himself at a "B" for his exercise habits. During a heavy work schedule he will stop exercising at the gym for two to four weeks. However, by regularly monitoring his blood pressure at home and every three to four months at his doctor's office, he notices that when he stops exercising for more than two weeks, his blood pressure rises. He believes that checking his blood pressure "keeps me honest" and prompts him to return to the gym.

Well dressed and well spoken, Harvey is a 62-year-old married man and the founder of a successful marketing firm. Harvey came to the clinic for a second opinion about treatment of his hypertension. For more than 15 years, Harvey had been told his blood pressure was borderline but not high enough to need treatment. Several weeks before his appointment, he was placed on a medication—a beta blocker—to help control his blood pressure. Since taking this drug, he has felt tired much of the time and has lost his get up and go. Despite the fact that he was taking his medication faithfully, Harvey's blood pressure was still elevated (164/98 mm Hg). Also, he was beginning to acquire a dreaded side effect that he was most fearful of . . . impotence! Although he wanted his pressure to be down, he did not want his libido to go down with it.

It wasn't fair to have no energy, no sex, and no control of his hypertension. He wanted to be off drugs, but he did not want to have a heart attack or a stroke.

Harvey was switched to a calcium channel blocker (Table 8.3) Although he felt better, he became troubled with constipation at higher doses. An ACE inhibitor (Table 8.3) was added, but his blood pressure still remained elevated at 144/92 mm Hg. After having a normal exercise stress test, Harvey was referred to the YMCA adult exercise program. He began to jog on even days and lift weights on odd days, taking one day off each week. He met other exercisers and developed a close group of friends who encouraged each other. Through his involvement, Harvey's wife joined the program, too. His blood pressure dropped to the optimal level (122/80 mm Hg), and although he remained on two blood pressure medications, a third drug was avoided. Ten years later, Harvey continues to exercise regularly and combines this with the use of two low-dose drugs to normalize his blood pressure levels without unwanted side effects, such as impotence.

For years, Harvey had borderline hypertension or what is now considered to be high-normal blood pressure. High-normal pressure often results in hypertension as we grow older, especially if we don't alter lifestyle factors. The only risk factors for high blood pressure Harvey had were his lack of exercise and his age. Although he was unable to control his blood pressure without medication, by adding exercise to his prescription, he was able to lower the dose of the two drugs and manage his hypertension without drug side effects. Using lower doses of two or more medicines rather than high doses of one drug can reduce side effects.

Not everyone develops the side effects listed in Table 8.3. There are many people who take these medications without feeling any differently than they did before beginning treatment. However, we rarely find that people feel any better after taking drugs to lower blood pressure. Is it any wonder that so many people don't take blood pressure medications, when the best you can say about them is that you might not feel any worse than you do right now?

Food Choices That Help Lower Blood Pressure

Beyond limiting salt and alcohol, certain food choices enhance the effect of exercise (and medications) and can help treat hypertension. A diet that (1) contains low-fat dairy products (below 30 percent calories from fat), (2) is low in saturated fats (saturated fats are the kind that come from four-legged animals and are solid at room temperature), (3) is rich in vegetables and fruits, and (4) limits intake of red meat can help tip the scales in your favor and reduce your blood pressure.

Exercise as Treatment

Many studies involving different age groups and differing exercises have shown that regular physical activity lowers blood pressure for those who have hypertension. A review of over 20 physical activity and blood pressure studies showed that systolic blood pressure is lowered about 11 mm Hg and diastolic blood pressure is reduced an average of 8 mm Hg with regular exercise. These effects have been documented for men, women, and children and can occur after just a few weeks of training.

Lowering blood pressure 8 to 11 mm Hg is similar to the changes found after treatment with a typical blood pressure–lowering medication.

Reducing blood pressure to this degree can reduce stroke and heart attack rates by over 25 percent! So, exercise can be the difference between being placed on drugs, with all their possible side effects and cost, and not needing any other treatment. For others, exercise can eliminate the need for one or more blood pressure medicines.

Beyond blood pressure control, exercise helps you feel better, decreases other risks for heart and blood vessel disease, lowers body fat, and improves your fitness level. On the other hand, blood pressure medicines do none of those. And remember, the best they can do is not make you feel worse.

Kinds of Exercise That Lower Blood Pressure

Nearly all exercises lower blood pressure. Endurance exercises such as walking, jogging, swimming, stair climbing, and bike riding can help control blood pressure. Even weight lifting can be used to treat hypertension. Practically any physical exercise you can think of can be used to lower your blood pressure. However, to be effective and to improve your chance of success, you should select exercises you enjoy and that are convenient. To get some motivational tips, check out Chapter 2.

How Exercise Lowers Blood Pressure

Exercise appears to reduce blood pressure in several different ways. First, just taking off fat through physical activity will lower blood pressure; this is similar to reducing body fat by dieting. But exercise has several advantages over just dieting. Breathing more rapidly, even with low levels of exercise, and sweating during physical activity help you get rid of water and salt, as would using a diuretic to lower blood pressure. Also, exercise affects two major hormones in our body. With training, your resting level of adrenaline is reduced. This lowers your heart rate and blood pressure, just as if you used a beta blocker, but with several major differences. Using beta blockers causes you to become less fit (they typically reduce aerobic fitness by 10 percent), but exercise makes you more fit. Instead of feeling more fatigued and losing sleep, you have more energy and sleep much better. And importantly, the blood cholesterol and sugar abnormalities that can occur with beta blocker use do not occur, and your cholesterol levels and blood sugar handling are improved with exercise (see also Chapters 5 and 6).

Another hormone, insulin, which is made in our pancreas (see Chapter 5), circulates in our bloodstream and helps control sugar levels. Some people with hypertension have high circulating levels of insulin because of a condition referred to as insulin resistance. Their body needs to produce more insulin to control sugar. Although this condition most commonly occurs when we have too much body fat, it can occur for no apparent reason. These higher than usual insulin levels will increase our body's salt stores by making our kidneys hold on to sodium. This results in higher blood pressure. Regular exercise reduces insulin levels (see also Chapter 5), and this effect alone may reduce blood pressure.

How Hard Do I Need to Exercise?

No pain, no gain? As for blood pressure lowering, this is not the case. You don't need painful or even vigorous training to gain benefits. How do we know? We have experimental evidence from laboratory animals and humans. Studies show that rats and humans are alike in more ways than you might think. We all know that both rats and politicians will desert a sinking ship. But did you know that both humans and rats can reduce their blood pressure with only light physical activity? It's true. Lowering blood pressure by exercise is not related to how hard you work out. In fact, low levels of exercise have the same or even a better effect on blood pressure than more strenuous types of exertion. In a 1999 report of men who walked to work, high blood pressure was prevented when the daily walk was over twenty minutes.

For control of hypertension, just do some form of exercise for about 30 minutes, three to four times each week. So with just 90 minutes a week of physical activity, you can keep the blood pressure drugs (or at least their high doses) away.

Exercise Rx for Hypertension

Pre-Exercise Points

Chapter 12 discusses preparation for physical activity. But there are a few points that need to be emphasized for those with high blood pressure, or if you are being treated for hypertension. So, before you reach for running shoes, jump on the stair stepper, or grab a weight belt to begin your workout, discuss your exercise plans with your physician. During this appointment, other cardiovascular risk factors should be checked, and the effect of your blood pressure on your body can be evaluated. Any potential problems with the medicines you are presently taking need to be reviewed. This often means your appointment will include the taking of your medical history and a physical examination, blood tests, a urinalysis, and possibly an electrocardiogram. You may need an exercise stress test if you are a male and over 40 years old, or a female and over 50, have cardiovascular symptoms, or have two or more heart disease risk factors (see Chapter 9, pages 160–164). If your doctor is not up to speed on exercise, tell her or him to read the textbook *Exercise for Prevention and Treatment of Illness* by Linn Goldberg and Diane L. Elliot. Be sure to talk to your health care provider first and do not begin an exercise program if you answer yes to any of the questions in Chapter 1, Table 1.3.

How to Begin

If you are just starting out, it is very easy to begin by walking. Walking always gets you off on the right (or left) foot. But whatever you do, begin slowly. This is going to be a lifestyle, so choose a time of day, days of the week, and activities that work for you.

How Long Should I Exercise?

Start with just 20 minutes, (Table 8.4). You can split your physical activity into two 10 minute periods, if it is more convenient. Then add 2 minutes to each exercise day, every week, to reach a minimum of 30 minutes, three times each week.

TABLE 8.4   **Initial Formula for Exercise**

Type of exercise:	Aerobics or weight lifting (your choice)
Intensity (how hard):	65 to 75 percent of maximal heart rate, or perceived exertion level of 2 to 3 out of 10 for aerobics; for weight lifting, check out Chapter 12
Duration (how long):	20 minutes, increasing to 30 minutes
Frequency:	At least three times each week

However, just as some people require a larger dose of medicine to control their blood pressure, you may require a larger dose of exercise. We suggest increasing the number of exercise days, if this is the case. In any event, you will probably want to do this anyway, because exercise will make you feel so much better.

Choosing an Exercise

Select activities you like to do and that fit into the time constraints of your life. Don't worry about your skill level or how you will look. For example, if you select swimming, constant activity for 20 minutes is sufficient for the first two weeks. It doesn't matter how far you go or how well you can swim (if you are not a strong swimmer, make sure you can stand in the pool with your head out of the water). If you choose to ride a bike, try an exercycle (a stationary cycle). It is usually easier to use in the beginning, and unless you are climbing hills, your workout will be more efficient and probably more vigorous. With stationary bikes there is no starting and stopping at corners; you can't fall off, become lost, or get a flat tire. Please check Chapter 12 for exercise tips.

How Hard Should I Exercise?

You can use the guide in Table 8.4 to find your training heart rate during your workout. You only need to exercise at 65 to 75 percent of your maximum heart rate to lower blood pressure. If you are using a medicine that has changed your heart rate, you can use the convenient perceived exertion scale (Chapter 12, Table 12.4, page 233). On a scale of 0 to 10, where 0 represents the amount of exercise you get by relaxing on the couch and 10 is the most exercise you can do, you should exert yourself at a level of 2 to 3. By rating your own level of exertion, you don't have to rely on heart rates, which can be different from person to person and be altered by taking certain medications.

What Should I Do When I Use Blood-Pressure-Lowering Medication(s) and Want to Exercise?

Essentially, there are no reasons not to exercise when you are taking drugs to lower blood pressure. However, it is always necessary to check with your health care provider before you exercise, especially when you are taking medications, no matter what they are.

When you exercise while taking blood pressure–lowing drugs, it is often best to use the perceived exertion scale and rely less on heart rate formulas. Using your heart rate as a guide is not very helpful when you take medications such as beta blockers, certain central alpha agonists (like clonidine), or calcium channel blockers. There are some specific recommendations for certain blood pressure drugs. If you use diuretics, it is important that you receive enough potassium and magnesium to replace losses due to the drug and exercise. Beta blockers reduce endurance exercise capacity by lowering the heart rate, and through other effects. This characteristic is great for people with both coronary artery disease and high blood pressure because it allows exercise with reduced pain symptoms and lower blood pressure, resulting in less stress on the heart. Some vasodilator drugs can increase heart rates. Because of the possible drug effects on heart rate, and the possibility of miscalculation when you determine your training heart rate, using the perceived exertion scale is a better way to go.

How Long Will My Blood Pressure Stay Down after I Stop Exercising?

In one respect, exercise to treat blood pressure is much like using a medication. After you stop training, its effect slowly diminishes. In a study that looked at the question of exercise as therapy for hypertension, 54 people with high blood pressure exercised three times a week on an exercycle. After three months, average blood pressures dropped to the normal range. Then, 14 of the people who had become fit and lowered their blood pressure, abruptly stopped exercising. Three months later, their hypertension reappeared.

The bottom line is, if you decide to stop exercising, get on medication, or if you are already taking medicines to treat hypertension, have your blood pressure monitored in case you need to boost the dose.

Remember Sarah and her high blood pressure reading at the dentist office?

Sarah went to the clinic and found that she did indeed have hypertension. With the help of counseling and nicotine patches, she was able to stop smoking. Her dietary habits changed as well. She purchased only low-fat, high-fiber breads and cereals. Skim milk became the only milk in the house, since she learned the "low-fat" 2 percent variety has more than 37 percent of its calories from fat. She looked at fast food restaurant menus and discovered there were items she could choose, including chicken breast sandwiches (without the mayo, please), salads, and low-fat shakes. She limited high-fat foods, although she occasionally ate desserts while dining with friends. Importantly, she began parking one mile from her workplace and walked to and from work each day. Every Saturday and Sunday she walked $2^1/_2$ miles. Sarah gradually lost over 22 pounds, and her blood pressure dropped to 126/82 mm Hg, without using medications.

Sarah had smoking, excess body weight, a high-salt and high-fat diet, and lack of exercise as risk factors for developing high blood pressure. Although her children were active, she was not. By making a few changes in her diet such as drinking skim instead of 2 percent milk, eating a high-fiber and low-fat breakfast, making low-fat, fast food choices, and parking one mile away from her work, she was able to fit her lifestyle changes into her current activities, without missing a beat. Her walking alone burned 1,500 extra calories each week. This degree of activity burns about two pounds of fat each month. However, even without any fat loss, exercise can significantly reduce your blood pressure.

Final Message

Regular exercise reduces your chance of developing high blood pressure and can lower your blood pressure if you already have hypertension. Even low level physical activity can be very effective as a blood pressure treatment. Although not everyone will be able to avoid medication, most will be able to control their blood pressure with fewer drugs or lower doses. In addition to all of this, exercise reduces risk factors for other diseases and provides you with an incredible psychological boost.

Chapter 9

Exercise to Prevent and Treat Heart Disease

"I feel like there's a thousand pounds sitting on my chest." Donna, a 39-year-old civil engineer, sat with her posture frozen as she spoke to the doctor. She was afraid to move because of the pain. Donna's chest and upper back had been bothering her for about four days, but now the pain was becoming much worse. The pain increased when she inhaled a cigarette, and she said, "It never goes away, even when I rest."

Donna's father died at age 42, and his two brothers had died suddenly before the age of 50. Their deaths were presumed to be due to heart disease. Her mother was alive and well. Although Donna smoked, she never had high blood pressure and did not remember whether her cholesterol level had ever been checked.

After listening to Donna's heart and lungs with the stethescope, her doctor, also a woman, declared that the exam appeared normal. She was given an inhaler treatment to see if this was an attack of asthma, but that did not change her symptoms. Finally Donna was told that her complaints were probably due to a lung infection, and she was sent home with antibiotic samples and pain medication.

Fortunately, another physician diagnosed Donna's problem several hours later as an acute heart attack. Angioplasty and a coronary stent were a lifesaver for Donna. She quit smoking but has not given exercise a chance.

Peter turned to his wife and said slowly and deliberately, "Call 911." After a pleasant midafternoon sexual interlude at their beach condominium, Peter, a 62-year-old stockbroker, was having difficulty breathing and felt a knifelike pain in his back. Sweat was pouring off his forehead. He was not sure what was happening, but whatever it was, he was frightened.

The emergency medical service from the local fire department arrived within minutes, placed oxygen prongs in his nostrils, pasted sticky pads attached to wires on his chest, and plugged the wire tips into a portable heart monitor. He was quickly transported by ambulance to the community hospital. The emergency room physician told Peter he had a myocardial infarction (heart attack). After two days in the intensive care unit, he was transferred to the University Hospital for care.

Peter could not understand his predicament. He said, "I have aunts and uncles who are in their nineties, and my parents lived until their late eighties." His cholesterol count was normal (despite his passion for fried foods), he had never had high blood pressure, and he had not smoked since his early twenties. "How could this happen to me?" Peter's only exercise consisted of walking back and forth between his office and the parking lot five days a week. The problem was, the lot was just two blocks away from the office.

Determined to learn why he had a heart attack and to prevent any new ones, Peter asked questions about his risks and wondered whether he could engage in sexual activity without fearing another catastrophe. After looking at his old cholesterol test results, one problem stood out. His HDL cholesterol was very low at 26 mg/dL. Although his total cholesterol count was only 197 mg/dL, the ratio of total cholesterol to HDL cholesterol was over 7.5. This alone more than doubled his chance of developing heart disease. Add to these risks his lack of exercise and age, and Peter's chances of developing heart disease quadrupled! To find out more about his future risks required further study.

Peter began his exercise program in earnest. Now, 10 years later, he has shed 20 pounds, never has chest pain, and is in the best shape of his life. He exercises three to five days each week by jogging and doing occasional weight lifting. He does take aspirin, vitamin E, and a cholesterol-lowering medication. His sexual activity continues, without Viagra.

The average ratio of total cholesterol to HDL-cholesterol is approximately 4.5. Your risk for coronary heart disease doubles with a ratio of 7 or higher, while your chances are cut in half with a ratio of 3 or lower.

As a freelance writer, Ruth spent most of the day at her word processor. In the evening, she watched television, read, or went out with friends. She did little housework because she hired a local cleaning service to do this chore. At 58 years of age, Ruth had never done much exercise.

Over the last several years she had developed mildly elevated blood pressure (154/94 mm Hg), and her cholesterol levels became abnormal. Ruth's total cholesterol count was 284 mg/dL, but her HDL cholesterol level looked good at 66 mg/dL. Her problem was that her LDL cholesterol level (the bad cholesterol, the kind you don't want) was 196 mg/dL.

For men and women without coronary artery disease, the goal is to reduce LDL cholesterol below 130 mg/dL

There are many types of heart disease, including diseases of the heart valves, the muscle itself, and the arteries. The most common heart disease is coronary heart disease, which is a narrowing of the arteries that supply the heart with blood. This restriction is usually caused by a build-up of fatty "plaques" that are loaded with cholesterol. As the obstruction to blood flow becomes more severe, the heart becomes starved for oxygen and angina pectoris (chest pain) can result. A heart attack, or myocardial infarction, occurs when a clot forms over the plaque or when the fatty tissue peels off the artery wall, obstructing most or all of the blood flow.

One out of every two men and one out of every three women aged 40 and under will develop coronary heart disease.

Taking her doctor's advice, Ruth had an exercise stress test. After passing the test, she signed up to participate in the group exercise sessions at the University Hospital. She hoped to lose some of those 30 pounds she had put on over the past 10 years, as well as lower her cholesterol level and blood pressure. Ruth began by walking around the basketball court, listening to the music from the stereo system's speakers on the gym wall at 6 A.M. She started with three sessions each week, and by the fourth week, she had increased to five weekly sessions. After four weeks of training, she received weight-lifting instruction and began to pump some iron, using light weights. Each Monday, Wednesday, and Friday she lifted weights for 20 minutes after walking for 30 minutes. On Tuesday and Thursday, she walked the entire session or rode a stationary bike and watched the morning television news show. Ruth continues to exercise five days each week. Fifteen years after her first workout, she feels better, has gained a close friend and exercise partner, and has lost 15 pounds of unnecessary body fat. She has had no cardiovascular problems and appears younger than she did before she started exercising.

Are You at Risk for a Heart Attack?

Donna, Peter, and Ruth were at high risk for coronary heart disease, a condition of narrowed arteries that reduce blood flow to the heart. Despite those risks, Donna's first health care provider misdiagnosed her chest pain. Although she reported the same complaints to an emergency room physician just a few hours later, that doctor also failed to obtain an electrocardiogram or other laboratory studies. He told Donna to just continue taking the pain medication. It was not until Donna's visit to a third physician that she learned she had suffered a heart attack.

What was the problem in making the diagnosis for Donna? She had the symptoms of a heart attack (Table 9.1)—"chest pain" and "a thousand pounds sitting on my chest"—and risk factors for coronary heart disease were present (Table 9.2)—a family history of heart disease at a young age and cigarette smoking. What else did she need? The problem was that most people, including many physicians, expect men to have heart disease, not women. Young women don't have heart attacks . . . right? Wrong! Sometimes heart attacks are missed because there are no symptoms, but many times the symptoms for women are different or, as in Donna's case, unexpected.

TABLE 9.1	**Common Heart Attack Symptoms**

Chest pain
Jaw and/or arm pain
Sweating
Nausea
Vomiting
Shortness of breath
Feeling anxious
Dizziness/light-headed feeling

According to a study done by the Washington, D.C., Hospital Center, twice as many primary care doctors believe breast cancer, rather than heart disease, is a greater risk to women. Despite their beliefs, cardiovascular diseases are the number-one killers of women, resulting in over 500,000 deaths each year, while during the same period, breast cancer claims the lives of about 43,000 women. Should Donna have suspected she had heart disease? According to the American Heart Association, only 8 percent of women in the United States consider heart disease and stroke to be the greatest threat to their health.

Besides the fact that many patients and physicians are not aware of the amount of heart disease among women, some of the warning signs may be different. Rather than chest pain, which is a predominant symptom among men, women may have nausea, dizziness and fatigue, or shortness of breath as their main symptom.

Approximately 240,000 women die each year of heart disease alone; this is five times more deaths than from breast cancer. Approximately 45 percent of all female deaths are due to cardiovascular (strokes, blood vessel, and heart disease) problems.

TABLE 9.2	**Major Heart Disease Risk Factors**

Family history of heart disease
Lack of exercise
Cigarette smoking
Obesity
High blood pressure
Abnormal cholesterol levels
Diabetes

Heart disease is the number-one cause of death, both for men and women, in the United States. Each year 1.5 million heart attacks occur, and 25 percent of those end fatally. Millions of other men and women suffer from disabilities caused by heart disease. The major factors that increase your risk of building fatty cholesterol deposits in the arteries of your heart are listed in Table 9.2. For each one of these risk factors, your chances of developing coronary arteries that are hardened with fat and cholesterol plaques are increased. When you have two or more major risk factors, your chances of developing coronary heart disease become very high.

You can lower your chances of a heart attack and stroke (brain attack) by learning about and lowering your own risk factors. Take the test in Table 9.3 to find out your chance of developing heart disease. No chart is perfect, so the points and your total score are only an estimate of your risk.

The pain of a heart attack is most commonly described as a crushing, heavy, or squeezing feeling in the center of the chest. About one-third of the time, the pain can be felt radiating down the left arm. About one out of five heart attacks is painless.

Angina Pectoris

For many, a heart attack may be the first symptom of a heart disease. Others suffer with episodes of chest discomfort, referred to as angina pectoris (chest pain), before there is any permanent injury to their heart. The discomfort of angina pectoris is usually described as a feeling of pressure under the breastbone (sternum). Some say it feels less like a pain and more like indigestion. In fact, angina is often confused with other problems in the chest, such as lung infections (bronchitis and pneumonia), heartburn, and pain in the muscles or bones of the chest. Occasionally, angina may be recognized only as a pain in the region of the neck, jaw, shoulder, or arm, and not in the chest at all.

Angina pectoris is caused when your heart does not receive enough oxygen. But unlike a heart attack, the problem is reversible. The condition most often occurs when your heart needs extra blood flow because your heart rate speeds up, your blood pressure climbs, or both. If the coronary arteries are too narrow, they cannot deliver enough oxygen to the heart muscle, and you get angina. Exercise, emotional stress, or just a heavy meal can raise both your heart rate and blood pressure. The more narrowed the coronary arteries, the less stress needed to cause symptoms. The symptoms of angina last up to a few minutes. As heart rate and blood pressure fall, the pain is relieved.

The American Heart Association states that a lack of regular physical activity is responsible for 250,000 deaths in the United States each year.

Nearly 7 million Americans have angina pectoris.

TABLE 9.3 **Your Risk of Developing Heart Disease**

Answer each question

How Old Are You? Points

Are you older than 45 (men) or 55 (women)? One point for yes _____

Do You Have a Family History of Heart Disease?

Did your father have a heart attack before age 55? Two points for yes _____
Did your mother have a heart attack before 65? Two points for yes _____
Did your brother have a heart attack before age 55? One point for yes _____
Did your sister have a heart attack before age 65? One point for yes _____
Has a family member (father, mother, sister, or brother One point for yes _____
   had a stroke (brain attack)?

Your Smoking History

Do you currently smoke? One point for yes _____
Do you smoke more than 10 cigarettes each day? One point for yes _____
Have you smoked for 10 or more years? One point for yes _____
Do people you work or live with smoke in your presence? One point for yes _____

Your Cholesterol

Is your total cholesterol 240 mg/dL or higher? One point for yes _____
Is your LDL-cholesterol above 130? One point for yes _____
Is your LDL-cholesterol above 160? One point for yes _____
Is your LDL-cholesterol above 190 mg/dL? One point for yes _____
Is your HDL-cholesterol below 35 mg/dL? Three points for yes _____
Is your LDL-cholesterol below 100 mg/dL? Subtract one point for yes _____
Is your HDL-cholesterol above 75? Subtract one point for yes _____
Is your triglyceride level over 500 mg/dL? One point for yes _____

Your Exercise History

I exercise less than once each week. Add two points for yes _____
I exercise once each week. Subtract one point for yes _____
I exercise two to three times each week. Subtract another point for yes _____
I exercise more than three times each week. Subtract another point for yes _____

Your Blood Pressure History

My blood pressure is over 140/90 Add two points for yes _____
My blood pressure is over 160/105 Add another point for yes _____
My blood pressure is over 200/115 Add another point for yes _____

TABLE 9.3   **Your Risk of Developing Heart Disease** (*continued*)

Your Body Fat History

My weight is normal	Pat yourself on the back (but no points)
I am more than 20 pounds overweight	Add one point for yes _____
I am more than 50 pounds overweight	Add another point for yes _____
I am more than 100 pounds overweight	Add another point for yes _____

My Blood Sugar

I have diabetes or use medicine to control my blood sugar.	Add four points for yes _____
	Add up your points _____

Scoring

Below 2 = very low risk; 3–6 = low risk; 7–10 = average risk; 11–14 = moderate risk; 15–18 = high risk; 19–22 = very high risk; 23+ = call 911.

Unstable Angina

Typically, angina pectoris requires a certain level of stress that results in pain, whereas removal of that stress, or treatment, relieves the pain. This condition is referred to as stable angina. When the usual pattern of angina significantly worsens, or becomes unstable, it can signal an impending heart attack. Unstable angina occurs when the pain becomes more frequent, is not easily relieved by rest or medication, when it occurs at rest, or when the discomfort becomes more intense. Unstable angina is a medical emergency, and hospitalization is necessary.

The Risk Factors

Smoking

The Virginia Slims woman has really come a long way . . . she gets the same tragic, self-inflicted diseases as the Marlboro man. Most of the devastation is due to cardiovascular disease, including heart attacks and strokes. However, millions of Americans have suffered with chronic lung disease and various cancers due to use of tobacco products. Cigarette smoking causes more than 400,000 deaths per year in the United States. This means that in the next hour, another 45 Americans will die just because of their smoking habit. Even with all the antitobacco messages and widespread information about the risks of smoking, each day 3,000 new recruits in the United States (more than one every 30 seconds) begin the smoking habit.

The longer you smoke and the more cigarettes you use, the greater your risk for disease. The risk increases for people who live with smokers, too. In the end, it seems you hurt the ones you love: passive smoke increases disability and death among children of smokers. The good news is that it is almost never too late to stop. Even when long-time smokers quit, their risk immediately starts to recede. This can prevent their life from going up in smoke.

Your air supply is reduced with smoking. Besides all the death and disability, smoking limits your ability to exercise, even without lung disease. The carbon monoxide in smoke tightly attaches to your red blood cells and reduces your ability to use oxygen. Less oxygen results in lower endurance.

Hypertension

Chapter 8 covers the topic of hypertension, also known as high blood pressure. Your chance of developing cardiovascular disease (heart attacks and strokes) increases when your systolic blood pressure (the top number) is at or above 140 mm Hg, or the diastolic pressure (the bottom number) reaches or exceeds 90 mm Hg. Exercise reduces your chance of having high blood pressure, and if you already have hypertension, regular physical activity can knock about 10 mmHg off your systolic and diastolic blood pressure. If you already take several medications, exercise can reduce the dosage or the number of medications you need for treatment.

Exercise also improves many of the other cardiovascular risk factors listed in Table 9.2. In addition, participating in endurance exercise for about 30 minutes, three to four times each week will improve your aerobic fitness by about 25 percent, while your blood pressure drops.

A stroke occurs when blood flow to the brain is obstructed. This is usually due to the formation of a blood clot. Warning signs include numbness or weakness on one side of your body, difficulty speaking, or sudden blindness. There are approximately 600,000 strokes in the United States each year.

Cholesterol: Friends and Enemies of the Heart

Although cholesterol is not a true fat, it is certainly related to fat. The relationship is fairly straightforward. The more saturated fat (fat from four-legged animals) we eat, the higher our cholesterol level climbs.

Exercise can cut your chance of developing high blood pressure by 50 percent.

This is especially true for the harmful, artery choking, LDL cholesterol. Also known as the "bad cholesterol," LDL cholesterol builds up on the walls of our arteries, slowly squeezing off the blood supply. Because approximately 65 percent of our total cholesterol is LDL cholesterol, your total cholesterol count is related to your risk for coronary heart disease. So, physicians will tell you to keep your total cholesterol under 200 mg/dL, which usually means an LDL cholesterol below 130 mg/dL. For more information on cholesterol, see Chapter 6.

A Way to a Man's (or Woman's) Heart Is through the Stomach

One kind of exercise that lowers LDL cholesterol levels is weight lifting. In one of our studies, both men and women dropped their LDL cholesterol level after just four months of training!

You can lower your total and LDL cholesterol levels by limiting the amount of saturated fat you eat and by reducing the amount of fat you have on your body. Do this by keeping your fat calories at or below 30 percent of your total calories, while reducing your intake of saturated fat to less than 10 percent of your total calories. Also, your diet should contain no more than 300 mg of cholesterol each day. Studies have shown that the best way to naturally cut cholesterol levels is to combine exercise with a diet that is low in saturated fats.

Drugs, Vitamins, and Potions

Another way to lower your total and LDL cholesterol level is by using cholesterol-lowering treatments. These include nicotinic acid (also known as vitamin B-3), several types of drugs (referred to as statins), and the bile resins. Also, postmenopausal women can take estrogen, while both women and men of all ages can munch on . . . m-m-m good . . . fiber. Eating psyllium seed preparations or consuming other types of fiber—or just the bran in high-fiber cereals—can lower your LDL cholesterol level, too. Eating fiber and bran can reduce your amount of LDL cholesterol as much as 15 percent. Some of these therapies have side effects you may not want. Nicotinic acid, especially at the prescribed doses of 2 or 3 grams per day, can make you flush, cause gastrointestinal upset, and has the potential for toxic effects on the liver. Sound good so far? The bile resins (cholestyramine and colestipol) are not too appetizing. Besides tasting like beach sand, they can cause bloating, nausea, constipation, and abdominal discomfort, and they interfere with the absorption of other medicines you might be taking. The statins (lovastatin, simvastatin, atorvastatin, etc.) reduce the amount of cholesterol in your body by interfering with an enzyme in your liver that produces cholesterol. These drugs are probably the best tolerated, and we prescribe them more than other drug treatments. But statins may cause levels of liver enzymes to increase, resulting in a low-grade hepatitis, and some people develop gastrointestinal complaints. Another potential side effect in a few people is muscle weakness. A blood test for the muscle enzyme creatine phosphokinase (CPK) can determine whether this is a problem.

For women, the use of replacement estrogens after menopause can lower LDL cholesterol and raise HDL cholesterol levels.

HDL Cholesterol: Guardian of the Heart

You also have the good kind of cholesterol known as high-density lipoprotein (HDL) cholesterol. This cholesterol removes the fatty build-up from our arteries and carries harmful cholesterol back to the liver for destruction—sort of a chemical disposal system. The higher your HDL cholesterol level, the more protection you have from heart and blood vessel disease. When your HDL cholesterol count drops below 35mg/dL, your risk of coronary heart disease increases. Unfortunately, we cannot eat HDL cholesterol. Although some people are born with an HDL cholesterol spoon in their mouth because of favorable genetics, most of us have to earn higher HDL levels by exercising and/or losing body fat.

A moderate amount of alcohol can increase your HDL cholesterol level a few points and may even help prevent a first heart attack. But after a heart attack, researchers have shown that alcohol increases total cholesterol, LDL cholesterol, and triglyceride levels.

Triglycerides

Triglycerides are a storage form of fat (see Chapter 6 for more details). When your triglyceride level becomes elevated in your bloodstream, your chance of developing coronary heart disease is increased. One way triglycerides increase our risk of cholesterol plaque build-up in the heart's arteries is by squashing HDL cholesterol. The higher your triglyceride count, the lower your HDL cholesterol count. In addition to the risk of heart disease, very high triglyceride levels in our blood (over 1,000 mg/dL) can cause an inflammation of the pancreas (pancreatitis). This is a serious disease that often requires hospitalization and can result in long-term disability, diabetes, and even death.

Certain drugs are used to treat high levels of triglycerides. The drug gemfibrozil effectively lowers the triglyceride level by reducing our liver's production of this fat and blocking the breakdown of our fat stores. Along with this action, our HDL cholesterol level increases. It has been shown to be effective in reducing heart disease. Although it is fairly well tolerated, side effects occur and are mostly gastrointestinal, although muscle inflammation and weakness are a risk, similar to the statin drugs that lower cholesterol. Also, nicotinic acid can lower triglycerides when taken in high doses. Bile resins used to treat high cholesterol levels do not help. In fact, they can raise triglyceride levels.

Exercise and Triglycerides

Fat is a source of muscle energy. The body fat we store and the fat we eat are burned while we rest and as we exercise. Although carbohydrates are used for high-intensity exertion, triglycerides are more like a low-octane fuel, providing energy for lower-intensity activities such as walking, gardening, and jogging. About half of the calories we use when we jog come from fat. Exercise gets rid of triglycerides by using them up. In addition to improving fitness, physical activity supercharges our fat-busting enzymes and lowers triglyceride levels even more. As triglyceride levels fall, HDL cholesterol levels rise, and the risk of heart disease is reduced.

Diabetes

High blood sugar, or diabetes mellitus (also discussed in Chapter 5) is a risk factor for coronary heart disease and stroke. A major side effect of diabetes is that it silently accelerates the blood-vessel-narrowing processes and magnifies the harm of other risk factors.

Symptoms of diabetes may include excessive thirst, urination, and appetite. Some will develop a pins-and-needles sensation in their feet or hands, due to the effect diabetes has on the nervous system.

Children and young adults usually have Type 1, or insulin-dependent, diabetes mellitus. This is most often caused by the body's overactive immune system, which destroys the insulin-producing cells of the pancreas. Although exercise does not prevent Type 1 diabetes, it strengthens the power of the injected insulin, causing it to become more effective. So, those who use insulin will not need as much.

Women with diabetes have three to seven times the risk of coronary heart disease as nondiabetic women.

Type 2 diabetes is also known as non-insulin-dependent diabetes mellitus. This type of diabetes tends to occur in families and is most often related to not exercising and being overweight. Exercise can help eliminate this form of diabetes entirely, or reduce the need for blood-sugar-lowering medication. In fact, regular exercise may be able to eliminate 50 percent of the cases of Type 2 diabetes! No medication can do that.

Attack of the Body Fat

Some people believe they are too handsome for their height. Others may feel, "If only I were a little bit taller." This relates to being overweight, too. Approximately half of all Americans are overweight, based on the current definitions (also see Chapter 7). If we could trim some of the fat off our bodies (or grow very tall) and avoid obesity altogether, over 1 million people in the United States would not have coronary heart disease, and there would be approximately 150,000 fewer stroke victims each year.

Am I Too Heavy for My Height?

A convenient way to determine whether you are tall enough for your weight is to compute your body mass index (BMI). This index is computed by taking your body weight (in kilograms) and dividing it by your height in meters squared. Obesity is defined as having a BMI greater than 27.5 kg/m², while morbid obesity occurs when the BMI is more than 40 kg/m². To find your BMI, check page 126 (Table 7.3).

Does It Matter Where I Store My Fat?

The best place to store fat is in the cupboard of your kitchen cabinets, or maybe in your garage. Where you deposit body fat in your body has an impact on your risk of coronary heart disease, no matter what your other risks are. Those of us who store our body fat around the waist have greater health risks than those who tend to bank more fat around the thighs and buttocks. So, does that mean we use an abdominizer instead of a thighmaster? No, not really. Although this might sound like the right thing to do, we can't reduce fat on a particular part of our body just because we exercise that area. Sit-ups don't get rid of fat around your waist, and working your thighs will not concentrate the fat loss between your knees and hips. Where fat stores are used is based on our genetics. Some

To find out your fat storage risk, measure the circumference of your waist and your hips. Divide your waist measurement by your hip circumference (waist/hip). If your ratio is above .95 (men) or .85 (women), you are at greater risk.

people lose it first from the hips, some from the belly. Usually the fat around our waist is the first to go when we exercise and diet.

Do Diets Alone Work?

Few people are able to lose a significant number of fat pounds or maintain their weight loss unless they exercise. No matter what diet plan you use, exercise is essential to keeping the weight off. Let's repeat that one more time. Exercise is essential to keeping the weight off. If you do not exercise, the fat comes back, sometimes with a vengeance. So, 6 to 12 months after your diet, you may end up weighing even more than when you started. Why is this so? Our bodies are 40,000 years old. We don't have a twentieth-century or twenty-first-century model. These are the same bodies that suffered through famine and pestilence. So our bodies are sensitive to fluctuations in the food supply. As we reduce the amount of calories in our diet, our body begins to think it is starving. So, as it has for thousands of years, it goes into survival mode. Your metabolism slows down, and on top of that, you lose muscle. So, you become weaker and thinner. Later, when you allow this body to eat again, even when you eat less, it maintains its survival mode. Your metabolism is so slowed that your body tries to store much of the food you eat as fat, just in case there is another famine.

This situation can be combated by physical activity. Both aerobic exercise and weight lifting counteract the drop in your metabolic rate by preserving the amount of muscle you have. Importantly, you don't need to restrict calories as much, because you are burning them up with physical activity. Aerobic exercise burns the most calories over a given amount of time, while weight lifting builds more muscle. The more muscle you have, the greater your body's ability to burn calories, even at rest. A further benefit is the afterburn of exercise. When you train for 20 to 30 minutes, you continue to burn calories for another 30 minutes after you stop exercising.

What is important about weight loss and heart disease prevention is that the amount of weight you lose doesn't have to be large. Taking off just about 10 percent of your body weight can lower your risk of developing hypertension, abnormal cholesterol levels, and diabetes.

Exercise Prevents Heart Disease

No matter how it works, whether because of changes in risk factors or other benefits such as stimulating the clot-busting enzymes in your blood, nearly all studies show that regular exercise prevents heart disease. At the Centers for Disease Control in Atlanta, researchers closely evaluated over 40 studies concerned with exercise and heart disease. Not exercising was as harmful as having a high cholesterol level, developing high blood pressure, or smoking cigarettes. But since there are four times as many nonexercisers as there are people with high blood pressure or cholesterol problems, improving fitness in the United States would have a huge impact on the health of Americans. Table 9.4 lists several prominent studies that show the benefits of exercise in the prevention of heart disease.

Finnish scientists found that the amount of time you spend exercising is related to your chance of developing coronary heart disease. Those who exercise about 2 hours and 15 minutes each week cut their chance for a heart attack by more than half. Think of it, if you can exercise 34 minutes, four times each week, or 45 minutes, three times a week, you can substantially increase your chances of living a longer, heart-healthy life. Do you want to reduce your chances of a stroke? A 1999 report from Iceland found that people over age 40 who participated in low-level exercise, such as swimming and walking, reduced their chance of stroke by nearly 40 percent.

Exercise is not only good for the arteries of your heart, but also great for the arteries that supply blood to your brain. By just climbing stairs, dancing, walking, or riding a bike for 30 minutes each day, you will reduce your risk for stroke (a brain attack) by 24 percent. Exercise for an hour a day and you lower your risk by 50 percent!

TABLE 9.4 **Examples of Research Findings**			
Exercise Did What?	**How Many Subjects?**	**How Was Fitness Tested?**	**Author and Publisher**
Reduces the risk of heart disease by half.	2,779 men	Exercise testing	Peters and colleagues *JAMA*, 1983
Nearly three times less risk of death	4,275 men	Exercise testing	Ekelund and colleagues *N Engl J Med*, 1988
Eight to nine times less heart disease death risk	13,364 men and women	Exercise testing	Blair and colleagues *JAMA*, 1989
Less than half the risk of heart attack	1,453 men	Exercise testing	Lakka and colleagues *N Engl J Med*, 1994
Vigorous exercise protects men against death	17,321 men	Questionnaires	Lee, Paffenbarger and colleagues *JAMA*, 1995
Reduces the risk of stroke by nearly 40 percent	4,484 men	Questionnaires	Agnarrson and colleagues *Ann Intern Med*, 1999

Are You Ready to Put Your Heart into Exercise?

Are you ready to exercise? Does one part of you say yes, I really should begin and the other part say I'll have to start some day? Do you think you will start when you have less stress in your life? But will your life ever be stress free?

When you consider exercise, there are some questions you should think about, for example, how important to you is becoming more fit, and how confident are you in planning and participating in at least three exercise sessions each week?

If your answers are "not sure," read Chapter 2 to pump up your motivation. If your answers are more than "not sure" but less than "nothing can stop me," ask yourself why. But before you do, read on.

The Risks of Exercise on Your Heart

Although exercise has a multitude of benefits, physical exertion has the potential to trigger a heart attack or heart rhythm abnormality. When studies are done on people who have suffered a heart attack, about 5 percent say that their symptoms started right after vigorous exercise. Those who are at greatest risk of heart problems resulting from high levels of exertion are people who are sedentary. People who are better protected from the harmful effects of heavy exercise get regular exercise! And, the more days of the week you exercise, the lower your risk becomes.

Know your risk before you begin training. You can check your risk factors in Table 9.3 and answer the questions in Chapter 1, Table 1.3. Also, your health care provider can help you screen for potential problems by taking a medical history, giving you a physical exam, and seeing the results of some simple blood tests, such as a blood glucose (sugar) and cholesterol levels. We recommend an exam for all sedentary men age 45 and older, and all inactive women age 50 and older, even if you have no history of medical problems. Just think of it as a 45,000 to 50,000 mile maintenance check-up.

If you answer "yes" to any of the questions in Table 1.3, you need a medical examination no matter how old you are! If you are taking medications, speak to your doctor about exercise. Some drugs, such as beta blockers (propranalol, atenolol, metoprolol, etc.), slow your heart rate and lower blood pressure but actually can worsen your endurance. When people use beta blockers, it may make it more difficult to attain aerobic fitness. Other medicines, such as tricyclic compounds (amitriptyline, desipramine, nortriptyline, etc.) have effects that can cause dizziness and weakness and reduce your body's ability to sweat. Inability to sweat as much as you need during exercise can lead to heat illness (for more information, see the Afterword). Diuretics (water pills) can get rid of too much potassium and lead to irregular heart rhythms during physical activity.

After your physical exam, you can either start exercising, or you may be asked to have a further evaluation. One test involves taking your body out on the road to check out the fuel pump (your heart), the wheels and tires (your legs), and the engine (your muscles).

Stress Testing

A stress test is not indicated for everyone. This is especially true for those who are at low risk of heart disease or if you have been exercising without problems. The reason? No test is perfect. When people have no symptoms and have few risk factors for heart disease, they are more likely to have a false-positive result. That means they don't have coronary artery problems, even though the stress test result suggests an abnormality. So when an abnormal result occurs, you become worried and are subjected to more expensive and sometimes riskier tests. However, if you (1) are at high risk for heart problems, (2) have symptoms of heart disease, or (3) are over 45 (men) or 50 (women) years old and have not exercised in years, a stress test is often recommended.

The stress test is a little like taking a car out for a drive. Imagine walking into an automobile showroom. You see a car you like—the headlights sparkle, and it has a price you can afford. You walk around the car, looking at the grill, checking under the hood, kicking a tire or two. You open and shut the doors and examine the interior. You like what you see. Would you buy that car without taking it on the road? Does it stall when you accelerate? Does it rattle at 55 miles per hour on the highway? Just looking at the car, you can't tell.

People are similar to cars in certain respects. Some look great. Their eyes seem to sparkle, they have white teeth, lots of hair, and nice clothes, but the arteries that supply blood to their heart are clogged with cholesterol plaques. You can't tell there is a problem until you hook them up to the electrocardiography machine and have them exercise. So, those with risk factors or symptoms of heart disease are often sent to the stress-testing laboratory. In Europe, a stationary bike is often used. In the United States, we are more likely to use a treadmill. It really makes no difference. The typical test is an EKG, or ECG, (electrocardiographic) stress test. If the test is positive, you may have another test, either a stress echocardiogram (an ultrasound of your heart as you exercise) or a stress thallium test (a nuclear medicine examination of the heart after exercise). If this test is abnormal, you might be sent to the cardiac catheterization laboratory, where a coronary angiogram (heart dye test) is performed.

The stress echocardiogram test allows observation of the pumping action of the heart while you exercise on a stationary bike. If the heart's motion is disturbed during exercise, it signifies restriction of blood flow to that area. Thallium is a weakly radioactive compound that is injected into the arm after exercise. Because of its special properties, thallium is distributed within the heart, where blood flow is greatest. It does not immediately accumulate in areas of restricted blood flow. If there is coronary artery blockage, that area of the heart does not take up much thallium right after exercise. About four hours later, you return to the laboratory and have a repeat scan. If the area of low thallium uptake is now filled with thallium, this means that the thallium slowly accumulated at the restricted flow site during the four-hour wait, and coronary artery disease is suspected.

Comparing the Tests

Your health care provider can help decide what kind of stress test is indicated. An EKG stress test can detect heart disease about 70 to 75 percent of the time . . . in men. The younger the man, the less likely it is that this test will detect coronary artery disease. For women under the age of 50 to 55, an exercise thallium or echocardiogram should be used if coronary artery disease is suspected, because of the high number of inaccurate EKG exercise tests. But, the greater the blood vessel narrowing and the more blood vessels affected, the more likely abnormalities will be detected. Although a normal EKG stress test for men and older women does not mean you have an absolute, 100 percent clean bill of health, the longer and harder you exercise, the more likely it is that you don't have significant coronary artery problems.

The stress echocardiogram and exercise thallium tests are better at detecting disease. If these test results are normal it is very likely you don't have coronary heart disease. So, why don't we just skip the EKG stress test and get the more accurate screening tests? The main reason is cost. The cost of a stress echocardiogram or exercise thallium test is about five to eight times the cost of an exercise EKG!

Don was a 44-year-old FBI agent who wanted a stress test. That's right, he asked us for a test. He said he had had an exercise EKG every two years when he lived in Washington, D.C., and wanted to see how his heart was doing. Don had no risk factors for coronary artery disease, and he exercised for over an hour each day without problems. We tried to convince him that he did not need the test. But, he kept insisting, and he may have promised to pay cash, or it may have been a slow week in the lab. For whatever reason, Don was scheduled for the exercise electrocardiogram.

He showed up ready for action: red and blue tank top, yellow fluorescent shorts, and the latest running shoes. His biceps were bulging from years of lifting weights. Don was the picture of health and fitness. He looked like a life-sized action figure. Don completed 9 minutes of the protocol when his EKG began to look abnormal. The test was stopped within the next 20 seconds and he was informed of the abnormality. He couldn't believe it and felt devastated. Although he was told that the test results were most likely a false-positive response, Don requested another test. The next day he showed up with a new tank top, shorts, and a different pair of high-tech shoes. Unfortunately, the results were no different, and Don felt even more devastated than before.

An exercise thallium test was completed two days later. To Don, it seemed like a month. The results? Another abnormal result. So a coronary angiogram (dye squirted into the coronary arteries to determine whether an obstruction actually is present) was performed. This time the result was "normal coronary arteries." No blockage. Don looked like he had won the lottery. The cost of the unnecessary stress test?: about $8,500. The EKG and the thallium tests were just a Fib for Mr. FBI.

We presented Don's case to a room full of cardiologists at a university heart conference. Before disclosing the angiogram results, we asked for a show of hands to see what our esteemed cardiology colleagues thought. Half of the group predicted that Don would have true coronary heart disease. The other half believed the test results were false-positives, and he did not have any artery obstruction. It was like flipping a coin. In any event, 10 years later, Don is doing well. Retired from the FBI, he continues to exercise. He has not asked for any more stress tests.

Exercise to Prevent Coronary Artery Disease

Putting variety into your exercise keeps it more interesting. You can select from a wide variety of activities, including walking, jogging, cycling, weight lifting, or using exercise machines (stair climbers, elliptical crosstrainers, simulated skiers) when you exercise to prevent coronary artery disease (Table 9.5); however, you need to know your personal prescription for exercise.

TABLE 9.5   **Exercise for Prevention and Treatment**

Condition	Intensity (How hard should I exercise?)	Duration (How long should I exercise?)	Frequency (How often should I exercise?)	Mode (What kind of exercise should I do?)
Hypertension	Mild to moderate rating of 2–3/10	30–60 minutes	Three to five times each week	Walking, biking, jogging, swimming, light weight lifting
Diabetes	Mild to moderate rating of 2–3/10	30–45 minutes	Seven days each week	All aerobics: walking, jogging, biking, swimming; weight lifting
High LDL or low HDL cholesterol	Moderate to high rating of 3–5/10	30–60 minutes	Four to seven days each week	Jogging, cycling, weight lifting, vigorous aerobics
Obesity	Mild to moderate rating of 2–3/10	30–40 minutes	Three, or better yet, seven days each week	All aerobics: walking, swimming, cycling, stair-climbing; light weight lifting.

How Hard Should I Exercise?

The intensity of your exertion is determined in part by the risk factors you intend to modify. To lower blood pressure, treat diabetes, or decrease body fat, you can exercise at a fairly low intensity. For example, if we use the Borg scale (Table 9.6), with 0 being at rest and 10 equal to the hardest you can exert yourself, you need to exercise at only a level 2 or 3 to achieve many of exercise's benefits. Training at this level, you are exercising at about 65 to 75 percent of your maximal heart rate.

To calculate your maximal heart rate (MHR), subtract your age from 220 or use the heart rate measured at the time of your stress test.

If you are trying to reduce your LDL cholesterol level or raise your HDL cholesterol level, you need to exercise more vigorously—at a level of 4 out of 10, 75 to 85 percent of your maximal heart rate. But no matter how hard you exercise, always warm up by training at a very low intensity and stretching to prepare your muscles and tendons for more vigorous exertion (also see Chapter 12).

Weight-lifting guidelines are not hard and fast; however, you should be able to lift a weight 10 to 12 times, for cardiovascular conditioning purposes. If you can lift a weight more than 20 times, it is not much of a strength-training exercise and won't build a lot of muscle, although it can improve your endurance. Fewer than six repetitions is not helpful from a cardiac standpoint. You can exercise all major

---

TABLE 9.6 **Your Perceived Exertion Scale***

Rating	What It Means
0	Nothing
1	Very weak
2	Weak
3	Moderate (I can still talk in full sentences)
4	Moderately strong
5	Strong
6	Stronger
7	Very strong
8	I am close to my maximum
9	I don't think I can do much more
10	Okay, I quit!

*Adapted from Borg GA: Med Sci Sports Exerc 14:377–387, 1982.

muscle groups (see Chapter 12) and train three times each week or split up your routine and exercise every day. You just don't want to train the same body part two days in a row. Your muscles need about 24 to 48 hours to repair and become stronger.

How Long Should I Exercise?

Plan about one-half hour of exercise at your perceived exertion level or training heart rate (see Chapter 12). Allow for about 5 minutes of warm-up before and about 5 minutes of cool-down after each session. When you start your aerobic program, you can begin with just 5 to 10 minutes of aerobic exertion and slowly build your endurance over several weeks or months. Remember, you want to be able to continue the exercise for years. Do not try to become fit in just a few days. It does not work. Take your time, you have years to condition your body.

Weight lifting should take you no more than one-half hour, if you are dividing your workout into six sessions each week and training half of your major muscle groups on any given day. If you do a total body workout with weights, it should take you about 45 minutes to complete your training.

In a study of people with coronary heart disease, weight lifting and stretching for 20 to 25 minutes prior to aerobic training increased strength, treadmill exercise time, and muscular endurance in addition to increasing muscle mass and reducing body fat.

How Many Times per Week?

The type of training determines the number of sessions you plan per week. For general aerobic conditioning, three to four sessions a week and 30 minutes for every training period will improve your fitness by about 25 percent within eight weeks. Exercise five to seven times each week, and you will become fitter even faster.

If your desire is to lose weight or you are treating diabetes, we suggest exercising every day. Metabolic problems such as being overweight (too many calories stored for your height) or having diabetes require consistency. You can treat or prevent high blood pressure with three to four exercise sessions each week. To lower total or LDL cholesterol levels or raise HDL cholesterol levels, four to seven sessions of exercise should be performed each week. To alter cholesterol levels, the more, the better! This is where higher intensity and more total exercise are needed for change.

Treating Coronary Heart Disease

Two important goals of treating coronary heart disease are the improvement of the quality of life and the improvement of the quantity of life. When an artery that is delivering blood to the heart is narrowed and causing problems, the solution may be to open up the blood vessel. The most dramatic method is a mechanical or surgical approach. That is, increasing blood flow by relieving the obstruction in narrowed arteries.

Coronary Angioplasty

One often-used procedure is coronary angioplasty. A small strawlike tube (a catheter) with a deflated balloon on its tip is inserted into the artery where the area of obstruction is located, and the balloon is inflated. The cholesterol plaque is squished and flattened by the balloon, much like your trash is smashed by your garbage compactor. This reopens the artery. Unfortunately, about 25 to 30 percent of the time, the widened artery becomes narrowed again within the next six months. Also, for about 2 out of 100 angioplasties, emergency bypass surgery is needed. Sometimes a stent (a wire mesh, semirigid tube) is inserted and is better able to keep the artery open. After stent placement, blood-thinning medication such as aspirin or coumadin is required. A newer procedure known as laser angioplasty vaporizes fatty plaques on the artery wall. Another technique uses a type of shaver, like a dental tool. This device grinds the cholesterol plaque into tiny particles. Following this, balloon angioplasty is performed. Angioplasty is often reserved for people who have only one involved vessel. Donna, the first patient in this chapter, had angioplasty with a stent inserted.

The cost of angioplasty is over $22,000.

Coronary Artery Bypass Grafts (the Cabbage)

Another common method to increase blood flow through obstructed coronary arteries is a procedure known as coronary artery bypass graft surgery, also called CABG (cabbage). This surgery redirects blood around the narrowed artery, thereby increasing the oxygen supply to the heart. Portions of the veins of your leg or an artery from your chest

The cost of coronary artery bypass surgery is approximately $45,000.

At age 52, talk show host David Letterman had a 5-vessel coronary bypass. His cholesterol level was reportedly above 650 mg/dL.

can be used as the graft. To do this, the sternum (breast bone) must be broken so that the surgeons have access to your heart. While this is taking place, another doctor will be surgically removing blood vessels from your own body (leg veins) or using your mammary artery so that the vessel can be fitted both above and below the blockage. Once the grafts have been attached you will have a new, improved path for blood to flow to the heart, effectively bypassing the clogged area.

Medical Treatment of Coronary Heart Disease

Not everyone has angioplasty or bypass surgery. Some people will reduce their chances of a heart attack or improve their symptoms with medications, diet, and vitamins, and of course, exercise. There are a number of medications that can help prevent heart attacks.

Aspirin, either 325 mg every other day or one low-dose (81 mg) tablet each day, can reduce heart attacks and death for people with coronary heart disease. Aspirin helps reduce the chance of a blood clot forming on a fatty plaque, inside the coronary artery. However, aspirin can irritate the stomach, and there is a risk of developing an ulcer.

Nitroglycerine reduces the symptoms of angina pectoris. It relaxes the veins in your body so that the blood pools in the newly dilated vessels, reducing the workload of your heart. Nitroglycerine comes in fast-acting tablets or sprays. You also can use longer-acting tablets and patches. The main problem with nitroglycerine is the headache, flushed feeling, and dizziness due to low blood pressure.

Beta blockers lower heart rate and blood pressure. This results in less need for oxygen by the heart. People with narrowed coronary arteries can do more physical activity when taking these drugs. In addition, beta blockers reduce the rate of heart attacks and sudden death.

ACE inhibitors, also known by their longer name, angiotensin-converting enzyme inhibitors, can help protect against damage to the heart when started soon after a heart attack or when there is evidence of heart failure and the heart becomes an ineffective pump. These medications are also effective at lowering blood pressure and may protect against kidney damage, especially among people who have diabetes.

Lipid-lowering medication can reduce coronary heart disease by up to 50 percent. The benefits are not only for people with very abnormal cholesterol levels, but even for those with cholesterol levels that are considered normal. These medications can reverse the plaque build-up on the walls of arteries.

Vitamin E is an antioxidant, which can help prevent damage to the inner surface of your heart's blood vessels. The way this may work is the following: when cholesterol interacts with oxygen, it becomes oxidized. This corrodes tissue, similar to iron rusting. The unstable oxygen molecules produced, called free radicals (not to be confused with radical groups of the late 1960s), not only harm the inner surface of blood vessels, they limit the ability of the arteries to dilate. This can result in less blood flow to the heart under stress. Use of vitamin E, at the recommended dose of 400 IU each day, has been shown to reduce heart attack rates.

Vitamin C may help restore the ability of the heart's blood vessels to dilate, even in the face of coronary artery disease with blockage of blood flow. Vitamin C is also an antioxidant, like vitamin E, and may cleanse the tissues of free radicals.

Folic acid is a vitamin that may help prevent heart disease by lowering blood levels of the amino acid homocysteine. Homocysteine has been linked to increased heart and blood vessel disease. Another vitamin, B-6, also lowers homocysteine levels. Although future studies are needed to determine their value, suggested doses of folic acid (400 mcg) and vitamin B-6 (3 mg) that have this effect are higher than the current daily recommended dietary allowance (RDA) for these vitamins.

Cardiac Rehabilitation

Today, 7 million people in the United States have angina pectoris, nearly 5 million have damaged heart muscle that has lead to heart failure, and almost 1 million Americans survive heart attacks each year. Almost 600,000 Americans undergo coronary angioplasty or bypass procedures per year, while another 2,000 people have heart transplants.

An estimated 13.5 million Americans have coronary heart disease.

People who take part in a comprehensive cardiac rehabilitation program can greatly reduce the consequences of having coronary heart disease. These programs can limit physical disability, reduce the risk of a second heart attack and death, and help you resume a normal life. Doctors, nurses, exercise physiologists, and dieticians are the personnel that help guide these programs. At the core of every well-designed cardiac rehabilitation program is exercise. Usually there are three phases for people who have been hospitalized for heart disease, whether or not they have had any surgical heart procedure. Those who should enter these programs are listed in Table 9.7, while examples of the many benefits of these programs are shown in Table 9.8.

The Three Phases of Mending Your Heart

There are three phases of cardiac rehabilitation. As you progress through each stage, you will learn how your body responds to exercise, while improving your fitness and health. Your heart, lungs, and muscles of your body will become stronger, your risk of heart problems will be reduced, and you will be able to do daily activities with less effort.

Phase One

After a heart attack, CABG surgery, angioplasty, or angina, the first phase (phase 1) is during your hospitalization. Exercise is gradually introduced, often with the help of a stress test, to help you and your health care provider understand your limits to exercise when you start out rehabilitating your heart. During this phase, you are not going to be conditioned, but your body will be stimulated by activity and be ready to proceed to outside-the-hospital exercise.

TABLE 9.7 **Who Should Participate in Cardiac Rehabilitation?**

Participate in a cardiac rehabilitation program if you
- Have had a heart attack
- Are at high risk for heart disease
- Have stable chest discomfort (angina pectoris)
- Have heart failure
- Have had angioplasty, CABG, or other heart vessel procedures
- Have a pacemaker, implanted defibrillator, or heart irregularities

TABLE 9.8 **Benefits of Exercise after Heart Disease**

1. Reduces symptoms of angina pectoris
2. Improves symptoms of heart failure (breathlessness and fatigue)
3. Lengthens lives (reduces mortality by 25 percent)
4. Improves feeling of well-being
5. Lowers LDL cholesterol and triglyceride levels
6. Increases HDL cholesterol levels
7. Improves clot-busting ability of the blood
8. Improves strength and fitness

Phase Two

If you have had a heart attack or experienced cardiac surgery or angioplasty, you are at greater risk to develop heart rhythm disturbances, angina pectoris, and shortness of breath with exercise. Because of this, we recommend monitored exercise sessions where emergency assistance is immediately available. This is often available at hospitals or local community centers that have doctors and cardiac nurses on the staff. In smaller communities where cardiac rehabilitation classes are not available, home exercise can be done safely, as long as periodic monitoring by means of medical history, physical exams, and stress tests is performed to guide your exercise.

Phase 2 programs should follow the exercise principles in Table 9.9. But remember, these are only estimates of your workout schedule. Your prescription may vary, based on your health care provider's evaluation and stress test results.

TABLE 9.9 **Phase 2 Exercise Prescription**

- Intensity: 2 out of 10 (Borg scale); heart rate 65 to 70 percent of maximum, or based on ECG stress test
- Duration: Start with 10 minutes, increase 1 to 2 minutes per session
- Frequency: Three to five sessions each week
- Progress review each week; adjust the prescription with help from your health care provider

The goal of phase 2 exercise is to begin getting you into better physical condition, safely. In a monitored setting, your heart rate may be checked before, during, and after exercise. Your blood pressure should be checked at least before and after you have exercised. Some people who have a very low exercise capacity based on their stress test will have telemetry (monitored exercise throughout the session) and blood pressure checks at intervals, because they are at higher risk.

Most phase 2 programs last from several weeks to about three months. A wide variety of exercises are available, including walking, jogging, stationary biking, swimming, rowing, and light weight lifting. After phase 2, you are stronger and have more endurance and confidence in your abilities. Now you are ready for phase 3.

Phase Three

By the time you get to phase 3, you should be familiar with your body's exercise ability. Likewise, your health care providers should be confident that your heart disease is stable and you have the ability to self-regulate your own training. That means you know your target heart rate or perceived exertion level (from 1 to 10), how long you should exercise, how often you need to train, when you should increase the amount of exercise, and which types of exercise are safe for you. If you don't know, you are not ready to exercise at home.

After having established a base of fitness during phase 2, you build on your gains during phase 3. Although most people can exercise on their own without problems, organized programs are preferred for people at higher risk. The community rehabilitation programs cost about $3 per session. Importantly, they are very safe. An analysis of 157 cardiac programs reported only one fatality per 783,972 patient-hours of exercise. A number of insurance companies' benefits include cardiac exercise programs, because they know that people with cardiovascular disease who exercise regularly experience fewer cardiac problems and save the company health care dollars. Table 9.10 identifies some of the factors that let you know that it is safe to exercise on your own.

For all people with heart disease who exercise, a yearly stress test is necessary to set new goals and establish the safety of your program. If symptoms of heart problems develop, an evaluation by your health care practitioner is necessary. To increase the safety of your exercise program, follow the rules in Table 9.11.

TABLE 9.10 **Lower Cardiac Risk**

- Normal blood pressure at rest (below 135/85 mm Hg)
- Normal blood pressure and heart rate response to exercise
- Normal or unchanged ECG at the prescribed level of exercise
- Stable angina pectoris or no chest pain at all during exercise
- You can exercise about 5 METs* (walking 2 miles/hour up a 10 percent grade, walking 3 miles/hour up a 5 percent grade, or equivalent work) (see pages 231–235)

One MET (metabolic equivalent unit) is the amount of oxygen we use at rest (3.5 mL of oxygen/kg of your body weight per minute). Exercise capacity is often based on this measure.

Pumping Iron: Will It Help My Heart Pump Too?

About 20 years ago, pumping iron was a no-no for people with heart disease. "Too much stress," "the wrong kind of stress," "it damages your heart," were the responses of many physicians. Today we know that weight training can be great for protecting your heart, if it is done correctly (see Chapter 12). Weight lifting, also called resistance training, can lower LDL cholesterol levels, decrease blood pressure, keep your resting fat-burning metabolism up, strengthen your bones, and aid coordination. Upper-limb strength gains are especially helpful and protect your heart during lifting and carrying activities.

TABLE 9.11 **Safety Rules**

- Always warm up and stretch before you train.
- Avoid extreme heat or cold weather.
- Train regularly. Do not become a weekend warrior.
- Avoid overexertion, and stay within your limits.
- Report any symptoms of chest pain, arm pain, lightheadedness, or other symptoms related to your exercise.
- Always cool down after exercise. Keep moving for about five minutes before you quit.

Similar restrictions to vigorous aerobic exercise (jogging, cycling, swimming, etc.) apply to weight lifting when you have heart disease. You should have stable cardiac disease, without uncontrolled blood pressure, heart rate and rhythm disturbances, or angina. Never lift weights without clearance from your health care provider and cardiac rehabilitation instructors. In fact, always begin weight training under the watchful eye of a skilled instructor and in a cardiac rehabilitation setting. Lighter weights are preferred because they result in less elevation of your blood pressure during exercise. So, choose a weight you can comfortably lift 12 to 15 times. Progress slowly (see guidelines in Chapter 12, pages 235–246).

Chapter 10

Exercise to Slow (and Reverse) Aging

Like a metronome, her arms propelled her through the water, lap after lap. Kerri is a 74-year-young retired university professor, and she swims daily, logging 40 laps in a local pool. Although retired, Kerri still maintains a busy schedule of teaching and research. Over the years, her only need for physicians was for routine health maintenance care and the occasional sore throat. Twenty years ago, when having hot flashes, she began replacement estrogen and progesterone therapy, and for the last two years, she has taken medication for mild hypertension.

"Me and my car get checked out once a year," Tom told the clinic nurse, "and today is the day." Tom is 71 years old and about to compete in the 1998 Masters World Games. Tom was a good high school athlete and played intramural sports in college, but it was not until he retired and could devote more time to training that his abilities really blossomed. In his words, "I'm about as good a senior athlete as there is around here." Watching a 70-year-old marathoner on TV had inspired Tom to get serious about running. Now, he walks or jogs three miles each day, and he is an honorary member of a high school track team, training with them each spring. Tom records how far he runs and pretends he is jogging to visit one of his daughters, charting his progress on a big map of the United States.

We could have chosen many other examples like Kerri and Tom, women and men in their seventies, eighties, and nineties, who are healthy and vigorous. The elderly are the fastest-growing age group in our population, and many are aging well and enjoying life—the hale and not the frail elderly.

Our criteria for what constitutes elderly keep changing, the older we get. Like most baby boomers, our heels are dug in firmly, as we try to hold off the aging process. Advances in public health and medical care have allowed us to live longer, and all our life expectancies keep going up. Because of living longer, the proportion of those who are elderly has climbed. In the last 100 years, while the number of U.S. citizens has tripled, the number of elderly individuals in the population has gone up 11-fold. Today, you can expect to live at least 30 years longer than you would have a century ago. Of all the people who have ever lived to be older than age 65, half are alive now. Most of those over age 65 have no disabilities and say their health is good or excellent.

People who stay vigorous and healthy as they get older are said to be aging well. The MacArthur Study of Aging in America examined the factors that lead to successful aging. To their surprise, researchers found that choosing the right lifestyle is more important than having the right parents. In their book, *Successful Aging*, Rowe and Kahn list three things you can do to make the most of your later years. First, you need to avoid illness. Second is to maintain your mental and physical abilities. And the third component is to stay engaged with life. Exercise positively affects all three of those dimensions.

It is easiest to understand how regular physical activity helps maintain your physical abilities. Endurance, strength, and flexibility are all benefitted by exercise. Physical activity also helps avoid illness. The risk of many medical problems goes up as we get older. By the time we are above age 65, half of us will have arthritis, and one-third will have hypertension or heart disease. Those are two of the many medical conditions prevented and treated by exercise (as you can read in this book's other chapters). And physical activity is a means to enhance your engagement with life. Walking clubs, dance classes, and senior fitness programs are just a few of the ways exercise lets you learn new skills and interact with people of all ages.

In August 1998, the Fourth World Masters Games were held in Portland, Oregon, and 11,000 athletes from more than 100 countries participated. The oldest woman was Viola Krahn, a 93-year-old diver, and the oldest man was 103-year-young Ben Levinson, who won the shot-put competition for his age group. Time to start training? The games are held every four years, and the next one is in Melbourne, Australia.

You've heard of the three ages of man: youth, aged, and 'you are looking wonderful.'—Cardinal Spellman

Old age isn't so bad when you consider the alternative.—Maurice Chevalier

Use It or Lose It

Tom likened himself to his car, and you might be wondering whether, as with a used car, it is better to have a vehicle with low milage. Why would you want to exercise? Won't physical activity just speed the wear and tear on your muscles and joints? It is an important question, and researchers have looked carefully at whether we benefit from exercise as we become older. The bottom line is that we *do* benefit, and the older we are the *more important* it is to be physically active. *Exercise can keep you young.* It is the closest thing we have to the fountain of youth.

As shown in Table 10.1, physical activity not only prevents, but reverses many aging changes. For example, as you get older, you lose muscle. By the time you collect your first social security check, your muscles will have shrunk by 20 percent. Losing muscle made sense back in the days of our prehistoric ancestors from Chapter 1. In ancient times, as you aged, it became more difficult to hunt and gather food. To get by on fewer mammoth burgers, your body lightened its load, and muscle was lost.

These days, no one wants to lose muscle. Less muscle means your endurance drops, and you become weaker. Less muscle has additional effects that might not be so obvious. As your muscles shrink, your metabolism slows. Muscles are the part of your body that burns most of your calories. The more muscle you have, the more calories you burn. Loss of muscle and a slower metabolism are why we tend to gain weight each decade, (see the discussion on metabolic rate in Chapter 7, pages 127–129). The only way you can prevent muscle loss is with regular physical activity. With exercise, you can maintain your muscle size and are less likely to put on the fat around your belt line that so often goes with middle age.

As you get older, your joints stiffen. Older muscles lose some of their elasticity and resilience. They become like a cold rubber band, more likely to snap if pulled. And, like that rubber band, if your muscles are warmed up and stretched gradually, they can perform well. Regular stretching will keep you more flexible and reduce your chance of injury. Aging bones of both women and men lose calcium and become weaker, making them more prone to breaking. Regular weight-bearing exercise (along with enough calcium) prevents the gradual decline in bone strength that would otherwise accompany aging (see also Chapter 3 on bone health).

The American College of Sports Medicine (ACSM) is a national organization of doctors, research scientists, fitness instructors, physiologists, and others involved in exercise and sports. In 1998, experts from the ACSM looked critically at all the research on exercise and aging. They summarized their findings by saying "physical activity programs in

Fewer than one in five older adults gets regular physical activity. Many wrongly believe that they are too old to exercise and sit back in their easy chairs. Facts are that as you get older, it's good to be out and about and "off your rocker."

I don't want to achieve immortality through my work. I want to achieve it through not dying.— Woody Allen

Older muscles respond more slowly to training and are more likely to be injured. If you are in your twenties and inactive, then it takes about 6 months to get in top shape. After age 30, you can add another month for each of the years you have not exercised. Using that formula, if you are 60 years old and have been inactive for 30 years, your muscles will be making improvements for 3 years (6 months + 30 months = 36 months).

TABLE 10.1   **Exercise Prevents and Reverses the Aging Process**

Health Aspect*	As You Get Older	If You Exercise	Comments
Muscle tissue	↓ (decreases 20% by age 65)	↑	Regular physical activity prevents muscle loss and can build more muscle.
Endurance	↓ (decreases 10% each decade)	↑	Young and old muscles respond to training in the same way. It just takes older muscles longer to make the changes.
Strength	↓ (decreases 20% by age 60)	↑	
Heart attacks	↑ (increased chance of heart attacks and death)	↓	Being active at any age reduces your risk of a heart attack by 50%.
Bones	↓ (weaker bones)	↑ (stronger bones)	Weight-bearing exercise prevents bone loss and can increase your skeleton's strength.
Joints	↑ (degenerative joint disease, i.e., more wear-and-tear arthritis)	↓	Rather than wearing joints out faster, exercise strengthens your muscles, which protects your joints and reduces joint pain.
Body fat	↑	↓	Exercise prevents muscle loss and slowing of your metabolic rate, which can keep you from gaining body fat.
Fasting blood sugar levels	↑	↓	Regular exercisers are half as likely to develop diabetes, and for those with diabetes, blood sugar control is improved with physical activity.
Flexibility	↓	↑	Losing flexibility increases your chance of injury. Stretching is an important component of regular exercise.
Blood pressure	↑	↓	Exercise can prevent hypertension, and low-intensity physical activities are all you need to lower your blood pressure.
Reflexes and coordination	↓	↑	To reduce falls, your exercise program should have activities that improve your coordination and balance.
Mood	↓ (more than 15% of the elderly are depressed)	↑	Studies of elderly living in the community and those in nursing homes find that regular physical activity increases peoples' sense of well-being, with less depression and more self-confidence.
Sleeping	↓ (insomnia and poor sleep)	↑ (improves sleeping)	People who exercise fall asleep easier and sleep longer.

*Many topics in this table (heart disease, hypertension, diabetes, osteoporosis, arthritis, and psychological benefits) are the subjects of other chapters in this book.

older adults may reduce the rate of age-associated deterioration in numerous physiological functions, . . . which in the long run, should benefit both quality and quantity of life." They recommended an exercise program that includes walking for endurance, strength training, and activities to maintain your coordination and balance. *Translation:* exercise keeps you young—it adds life to your years and years to your life.

Exercise and Menopause

Every woman who lives long enough will experience menopause, or the cessation of menses. In the United States, for most women, this occurs between the ages of 48 and 55. Menopause also can be brought on instantly by surgical removal of the ovaries.

Ovaries do not go from working normally to menopausal overnight. For up to a decade before menses stop completely, women experience perimenopause. Their ovaries are working, but less effectively. Menstrual cycles are irregular, and the fluctuations in female hormone levels are greater. That explains why symptoms of menopause can occur while a woman still has her periods.

Some of the considerations for and against estrogen replacement therapy (ERT) are listed in Table 10.2. Despite the fact that ERT has been available for more than 50 years, its precise risks and benefits are

Osteoporosis is an equal opportunity problem. Men's bones get weaker as they get older, just as women's bones do. One in five men older than age 65 will have a fracture due to osteoporosis.

TABLE 10.2   **Risks and Benefits of Estrogen Replacement Therapy**

Benefits	Risks
Relieves sysmptoms of estrogen withdrawal (vaginal dryness and hot flashes)	Eightfold increase in endometrial (uterine) cancer, unless estrogen is given with progesterone therapy
Reverses unfavorable lipid changes	May increase the risk of breast cancer
May reduce incidence of cardiovascular disease	Hassle and expense of taking medication
Preserves bone mass and prevents osteoporosis	Irregular bleeding, bloating, weight gain

By encouraging estrogen replacement therapy are we medicalizing a natural part of a woman's life cycle and diminishing the stereotype of aging individuals? By discouraging it are we denying women a health-enhancing hormone?

TABLE 10.3   **Effects of Exercise and Estrogen Replacement Therapy on Menopausal Changes**

Menopause Can Cause	Physical Activity	Estrogen Replacement Therapy (ERT)
Hot flashes	Hot flashes are less common among physically active women, although exercise does not uniformly relieve the problem.	ERT relieves hot flashes. Nonhormonal medications also are available to relieve hot flashes.
Disrupted sleep, irritability, mood swings, and depression	Exercise reduces feelings of depression and can improve sleeping.	ERT reduces feelings of depression and can improve sleeping.
Difficulty concentrating and memory loss	Exercise may increase alertness but probably does not affect your memory.	ERT may improve your memory for words and may delay (but not prevent) the onset of Alzheimer's disease.
Vaginal dryness	No effect	Relieved with ERT
Increased LDL cholesterol (bad cholesterol) levels and lowered HDL cholesterol (good cholesterol) levels	Exercise may help, especially by preventing a postmenopausal weight gain.	Adverse changes are reversed with ERT.
Increased risk for coronary artery disease (angina and heart attacks)	Regular exercise decreases the risk of heart disease.	Effects of ERT are not clear. Beginning ERT may increase your risk, while long-term use may decrease your risk.
Muscle loss and an increase in body fat, with an increase in abdominal obesity	Exercise burns calories and preserves your calorie-burning muscle mass.	ERT may prevent redistribution of body fat and development of abdominal obesity.
Loss in bone density and development of osteoporosis	Exercise (along with calcium and vitamin D) can maintain bone density.	Estrogen (along with calcium and vitamin D) prevents bone loss.

not known. The Women's Health Initiative study should give us answers to the effects of ERT. It is a huge project that includes more than 100,000 women with menopause who have been randomly assigned to different types of treatment—hormonal and nonhormonal—with careful recording of outcomes regarding breast cancer, heart disease, osteoporosis, and mental functioning. Unfortunately, we will not know the results until 2005. For now, each woman must weigh the pros and cons of ERT for herself.

The jury is out on hormone replacement therapy, but the verdict is clear for the benefits of exercise among women with menopause. Table 10.3 lists changes at menopause and the effects of exercise and ERT. Exercise counters most of the adverse effects of falling hormone levels, and unlike ERT, it decreases a woman's risk for breast cancer.

What Constitutes Exercise?

Today, Irene looks much younger than her 97 years. She lives independently in her own apartment, takes cabs to the grocery store, and has her hair done every other week. What is her secret? Hoping to have our bias about the benefits of physical activity confirmed, I asked Irene about whether she exercises. To my surprise, she said that her only exercise was as a youth. She recalled playing shortstop on a baseball team when she was in the ninth and tenth grades, and grass hockey in high school. After high school, she moved to a nearby large city and worked for a photographer for $3.00 a week. She said she stopped exercising. But additional questions revealed that Irene had walked four or five miles a day, going to and from work. Weekends were spent walking around the city's park, an acceptable place for young women and men to meet 80 years ago.

As do many people, Irene defined exercise as playing a sport or going to a gym. In truth, she had been exercising her entire life. Irene managed a restaurant until retiring in her eighties. During those years, she usually left her Cadillac parked in the driveway and preferred to walk to work. Even now, she has a daily stretching program and walks around her retirement complex, whenever the sidewalks are dry.

Some people think that exercise means playing sports and sweating. It is time to change that thinking. While you might not consider walking, climbing stairs, and gardening to be exercise, they are all physical activities. Your health improves when your muscles move, even if the movement is not what you would call exercise. Exercise is *any kind of physical activity* that contributes to your health.

For women, exercise can uncover incontinence, or leakage of urine. With lowered female hormone levels and aging, tissues in the pelvis become thinner, and the urinary sphincter weakens. You can strengthen your urinary sphincter and pelvic floor muscles with Kegel exercises. Squeeze the muscles that stop urine flow for one second, then relax for one second, completing that sequence 10 times. Gradually increase the number of contractions up to 30, and perform that sequence twice each day. Urination can be used to identify these muscles, but the exercises should not be performed at that time, because it might disrupt your normal voiding reflexes. Be patient with the process. It can take more than a month before you will notice an increase in urethral sphincter strength.

The Dangers of Rest

When at bed rest, your muscles lose about 2 percent of their strength each day. A month of being in bed can reduce your strength by more than 50 percent.

Carmela felt short of breath just walking across the room. Ten days of bed rest had caused her to lose strength and endurance. Still, she insisted that she could "get by at home" and did not want to go to a rehabilitation facility following her hospital stay. Carmela is 83 years old and recovering from surgery for colon cancer. The tumor was discovered when she developed an anemia. Her surgery went well, and there is a good chance she is cured. Unfortunately, she developed an allergy to one of her medications and had a rash over most of her body. The rash required her to take cortisone pills, which led to a high blood sugar level and a wound infection. Her hospital stay stretched to 10 days. Carmela was widowed six years ago and lives alone in an apartment. She has a daughter close by who wants to help, but Carmela is fiercely independent. She enjoys living alone and doing things for herself.

Many of the greatest benefits of exercise are enjoyed when your fitness level is the lowest. Figure 10.1 compares a person's physical fitness with his or her functional abilities. *Functional abilities* is a term that refers to activities that allow you to live independently, for example,

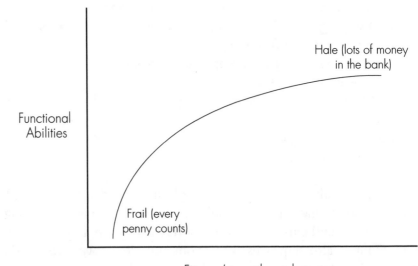

Figure 10.1   Fitness versus Function curve

getting in and out of a bathtub, climbing a few steps, carrying a bag of groceries, and making a bed. Your level of fitness is like your bank account. If you are Bill Gates and at the hale end of the curve, then a few more fitness dollars do not mean much. You have lots of fitness in the bank, and you could lose a billion or two credits and never notice the difference. At the other end of the curve, when your bank account is low, a little bit of fitness money can go a long way toward improving your life.

As we age, our natural tendency is to move down the curve, gradually losing fitness. At some point, we may hit the slippery slope, where our abilities really decline. At that end of the curve, if you lose just a little more strength, it can mean you are no longer able to do simple household chores or care for yourself. At the frail end of things, a little bit of fitness can keep you independent and doing activities that most of us take for granted.

It is never too late to pump iron. Even people in their nineties who have never lifted weights can get stronger by strength training. Researchers in Boston taught elderly men and women to lift weights. Although healthy, these seniors were weak. Before training, they could lift only 15 pounds with their thigh muscles, an amount that most people could easily lift with one arm. After just 10 weeks of exercise,

Nutrition and physical activity go hand-in-hand. Muscles need building blocks from protein for growth and repair. Older men and women should eat approximately 1 gram of protein for each 2 pounds of body weight. Studies say that more than half of the elderly do not get the recommended amount of protein. Table 10.4 lists high-protein foods.

TABLE 10.4 **High-Protein Foods**

Food	Calories	Grams of Protein
1 egg white	17	4
1 cup skim milk (8 oz.)	85	8
1 cup low-fat cottage cheese	163	28
1 cup beans and rice soup	150	9
1 cup Special K cereal	83	4
1 cup split pea soup	189	10
1/2 cup baked beans	280	12
1 cup low-fat fruit-flavored yogurt	223	10
1 Gardenburger patty	190	11
1 skinless chicken breast	141	27
3 oz. water-canned tuna	99	20
4 oz. light turkey meat	177	34

these former weaklings doubled their leg strength. That meant they could do more work without feeling fatigued. Their walking speeds increased, it was easier to climb stairs, and they were less likely to fall. Because of their new-found strength, they were more physically active throughout the day.

For the first few days after hospital discharge, Carmela's daughter spent the night in her mother's apartment. To help avoid falls, they installed grab bars and assistive equipment (for example, a raised toilet seat and a shower stool). A visiting nurse came by twice a week to monitor Carmela's wound, and a physical therapist began Carmela on a program to regain her strength and endurance. Although recovery took longer than she had anticipated, 18 months after her surgery, Carmela says she is back to her old self and feeling well.

Preexercise Check List

If you are older, especially if you have medical problems, talk with your health care provider before beginning regular exercise. Chapter12 lists guidelines to follow when you are beginning an exercise program. Be sure to mention it to your health care provider if your answers are "yes" to any of the questions in Chapter 1, Table 1.3. Your major risks from exercise and ways to avoid them are listed in Table 10.5.

What Kind of Exercise Is Best?

People beginning an exercise program usually want to know what kind of exercise is best. Your choice about how to exercise should be based on what you like to do and the physical benefits you want from exercise. Figure 10.2 provides a flow diagram to help match your needs with different types of physical activity. One of the first questions to ask yourself is how important socializing is for you. Would you rather be active with a group or exercise by yourself? For many of us, socializing is important. Remember that one of the three keys to successful aging

---

If you are older, to avoid injury and maximize the benefits of strength training, a program should be initiated with the supervision of a physical therapist or certified exercise trainer.

Preventing falls is important for the elderly. The most effective fall-prevention programs include endurance and strengthening exercises, plus activities that increase your balance. Tai Chi is a type of exercise that may be especially beneficial in increasing your coordination and preventing falls. It is discussed in Chapter 3, page 43.

TABLE 10.5 **Risks of Exercise for the Elderly**

Risk	How You Can Prevent It
Sore muscles and joints	Always warm up well before exercising. If you have arthritis or are especially concerned about this risk, select activities that cause less stress on your joints, such as swimming and water aerobics. Begin slowly and gradually increase your training. If you have joint problems, a physical therapist or certified trainer can provide advice about specific exercises to protect your joints.
Heart attack (see also discussion in Chapter 9, pages 160–164)	See your health care provider before beginning to train and immediately report any symptoms that might involve your heart (chest pain or pressure, feeling lightheaded, palpitations, or unusual shortness of breath). If you have heart problems, a cardiac rehabilitation program (described in Chapter 9, pages 181–186 may be best.
Injuries	When possible, do not exercise alone, and mornings are safer than evenings. Trust your instincts to avoid any situation that does not seem safe. If your safety while exercising alone is a concern, you can work out at home or in a community center. Use well-fitted, supportive shoes. Begin activities slowly and go at your own pace. Don't push yourself to keep up. "No pain, no gain" is not true!

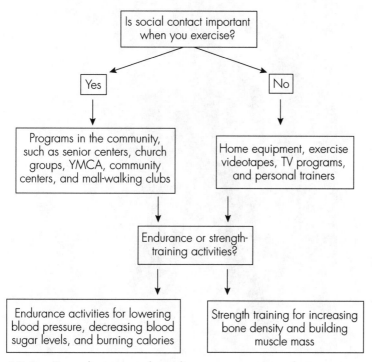

Figure 10.2   Considerations when choosing your type of exercise.

With some simple precautions, exercise is safe for all ages. When all the studies of exercise training among the frail elderly (ages 80 to 100 years) were compiled, none of the participants had sudden death or a heart attack while exercising.

is being actively engaged with life, and physical activity is one way to do that. Most communities have many opportunities for group activities—senior centers, the YMCA, and local recreation centers.

Sometimes transportation to a place for exercise is a problem. Or you may be concerned about your safety when out of your home and exercising. In those cases, you can exercise at home with the help of books, videotapes, and television programs geared for seniors.

It is best to have both endurance and strength-training activities in your exercise program. As shown in Figure 10.2, which one you choose might depend on the benefits you most want. During endurance or aerobic activities, your large muscles are used continuously, such as with walking, swimming, cycling, and dance. This type of exercise is

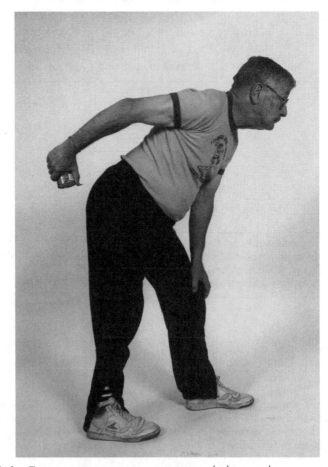

Figure 10.3   Triceps exercise using cans as a light weight.

best for burning calories, lowering blood pressure, preventing diabetes, and perhaps improving sleep. Strength training uses weights, springs, or resistance bands to make your muscles stronger. It increases your bone density, builds muscle tissue, helps prevent injuries, and speeds your metabolic rate. For the best results, your program should include both endurance activities and weight training, along with activities to increase your joint flexibility, coordination and balance. The tables in this chapter illustrate guidelines for a program of walking, water exercise, and strength training. Stretching routines are presented in Chapter 12, pages 246–256.

Your objective is to be more physically active throughout the day, not just to add in 30 minutes of exercise. It is ironic that as we get older, people start offering to carry our bags and give us a lift, when this is the time that doing things for ourselves becomes most important. One colleague said that his biggest mistake was starting to give his mother a ride to the store, so she did not have to walk. (We don't know how well it went when he told his mother that she needed to walk "for her own good.")

Strength Training

Strength training, resistive exercise, and pumping iron all refer to activities in which your muscles work against resistance. The resistance can be from your own body, elastic bands, springs, machine weights, or free weights. Like many sports, strength training has its own jargon, and weight-lifting terms are defined in Table 12.7. General advice about strength training is shown in Table 10.6, Exercises using light weights (Figures 10.3 and 10.4) or elastic bands (Figure 3.4 from Chapter 3 on bone health) can be used as you begin to strength train. Weight-training exercises using weight-training machines are described and illustrated in Chapter 12. Because of the potential for injury, learning proper technique and selecting appropriate weights are important. Initial instruction from a physical therapist or certified athletic trainer will reduce your chance of an injury.

Endurance Training

Endurance (also called aerobic) exercise involves continuous use of your large muscles. This type of training increases your heart and blood

---

TABLE 10.6   **Advice for Strength Training**

- Do not strength train the same muscles two days in a row.
- Your heart rate should slow down to near resting levels between sets.
- Begin with your larger muscle groups (such as your chest and back muscles) and save the biceps curls and other smaller muscles for last.
- Begin and end your workout with 5 to 10 minutes of walking at a slow pace and stretching exercises.
- Learn lifting skills before stressing your muscles with heavy weights.

Optimal endurance training is at a heart rate of 65 to 80 percent of your maximum heart rate. Your maximum heart rate equals 220 minus your age in years. For example, if you are 70, your maximum heart rate is 150, and your training zone is 95 to 120 beats a minute. To find your heart rate, check your pulse for 15 seconds and multiply by 4, or count 6 seconds and multiply by 10. When you are exercising, you should have enough breath to talk and be able to keep up your pace for more than 30 minutes without stopping. If you cannot do that, then you are working out too hard.

vessels' delivery of oxygen to your muscles, and it enhances your muscles' ability to use oxygen. Walking, swimming, cycling, and water aerobics are common types of endurance training.

Walking Program

Our muscles change at different rates. As we get older, things tend to take longer, and getting in shape is no exception. Though you might

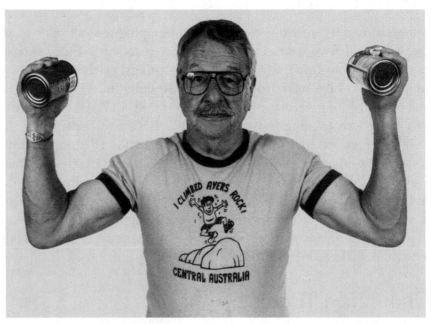

Figure 10.4   Light weights can be used to strengthen biceps and can be lifted overhead for the shoulder muscles.

not feel it, your body benefits *each* time you exercise. It takes months for younger muscles to get in shape, and older muscles can make gains for many months, with improvements occurring for more than a year. If you try to rush it, you will be risking an injury. If you are uncomfortable advancing at the recommended rate, *don't.*

Table 10.7 lists recommendations for a progressive walking program. The optimum intensity of endurance training is when your heart rate is 65 to 80 percent of your maximum heart rate. Although that heart rate might be best for conditioning your muscles to take up oxygen and increasing your endurance, less-intense physical activities (with a slower heart rate) may be just as good for burning calories, improving your coordination, lowering blood pressure, and improving your spirits. If it has been years since you last exercised, then starting slowly is best.

A safe place to walk and comfortable, supportive shoes are the only equipment you need for a walking program.

Water Aerobics

A pool can be used in several ways to add to your fitness program. Stretching exercises, calisthenics, and lap swimming are all activities done in the water. Because the water supports 90 percent of your weight, water activities put less stress on your joints. That is why water

		TABLE 10.7 **Walking Program**	
Week	**Workouts per Week**	**Walking Pace Intensity (you will know this by checking your heart rate)**	**Duration (minutes)**
1	2		15
3	3	About 60% of your maximum heart rate, a pace that you can comfortably continue for more than 30 minutes	15
5	3		20
7	3		20
9	3–4	65% of your maximum heart rate	20
10–20	3–4	65% of your maximum heart rate	30
21–28	4–5	70% of your maximum heart rate	30
29–36	4–5	70% of your maximum heart rate	45

TABLE 10.8	**Activities for Exercise in the Water**
Activity	**Description**
Walking	Brisk walking across the shallow end of the pool.
Running	Similar to walking, but take longer leaping steps and use your arms, or you can jog in place. Flotation belts will allow you to perform jogging in place in deeper waters.
Jumping jacks and can-can kicks	Perform these with your legs slightly bent. Kicks should not be too high.
Standing and stroking	While standing in chest-high water, perform these upper body movements. Cupping your hands will increase the resistance. Strokes to use include the crawl, breast stroke, and dog paddle.
Push up	Perform the exercise in chest-high water and lean against the wall.
Upper-body-supported lower body exercises	Lean against the wall, with both arms out at your sides and on the pool's edge. From this position, you can do exercises for your legs and midsection. Bend your knees with legs together, scissor your legs, spread your legs apart, and with your legs together, sweep them from side to side. The same movements can be performed away from the edge, if you hold a floatation device to your chest.

workouts are especially useful for those with arthritis or if you are very overweight. A program of lap swimming would be similar to the walking program in Table 10.7. Water aerobics usually combine exercises that increase your endurance, flexibility, and strength. Most are taught by an instructor certified for the activity and for water safety. You can design your own workout by putting together the exercises listed in Table 10.8.

Bottom Line

Physical activity is more important as we get older. Exercise prevents and reverses many of the adverse changes of aging. Most older women and men are healthy, and the general recommendations for training apply, with adjustments for their lower maximal heart rate and slower muscular response to regular exercise. Although activities must be modified, exercise is especially important for the frail elderly, because small increases in strength, endurance, and balance can have a big impact on their physical abilities.

Chapter 11

Exercise to Elevate Mood and Treat Anxiety and Depression

When asked about her mood, Cindy joked, "Some days, I feel like I'm going mental." Cindy was here for an annual exam, which she always scheduled for January. She complained of fatigue, of an increase in tension headaches, and of weight gain. Happily married in a two-career family, she found that money was always tight. When she was not at work, her children needed her to drive them to sports, band practice, and friends' houses. In addition, her aging parents depended on her for help. They were set in their ways and resisted her suggestions to move from their large two-story home into a more manageable one-level condominium. Cindy said that her long days were filled with one "have to" after another.

Cindy was concerned she might be depressed. She was having trouble sleeping, and she often felt down and tense. She wondered whether Prozac or St. John's Wort would help. We were in the middle of the short, dark days of an Oregon winter, but Cindy did not remember a pattern of her spirits being low at this time of the year. Although she felt down, she still found pleasure in many things and functioned well at home and in her work.

Physical Activity versus Prozac

Many of us lead stressful lives, and everyone has a few bad days. It can be difficult to know what is normal and if you are depressed. Depression is common and affects more than 17 million Americans. Its costs in treatment, disability, and lost productivity are comparable to the dollars spent on heart disease. The illness *depression* is more than just feeling down or sad for a day or two. With depression, those feelings

Depressed individuals sometimes ask themselves, "Why can't I buck up and get over feeling down?" The stigma of a mental illness and those thoughts can make people hesitant to get help for depression. Fortunately, that reluctance is less in recent years, in part, because of the many well-known people who have talked openly about their depression, for example, Buzz Aldrin, Art Buchwald, Dick Clark, Sheryl Crow, Jules Feiffer, Mariette Hartley, Bonnie Raitt, Joan Rivers, Rod Steiger, and Mike Wallace.

are with you most of the time and for longer than two weeks, and often you also lose interest or pleasure in all activities (Table 11.1). Nothing is fun anymore. It is difficult to think clearly, concentrate, and make decisions. You may have feelings of guilt and thoughts of suicide. Those symptoms are accompanied by changes in your sleep (either insomnia or sleeping more), reduced sex drive, and unintentional weight loss or gain. Many times, depression causes physical complaints such as fatigue, headaches, and abdominal pain. Although it may sound like depression is easy to recognize, at least half of its sufferers do not get proper treatment. You can fill out the Beck Depression Inventory in Table 11.2; this test is a standardized way to evaluate your own mood.

We do not know what causes depression. It tends to run in families, and in addition to genetics, life events and stressors play a role. However, depression can come out of the blue, when things are going well and you least expect to feel down. Antidepressants can dramatically relieve symptoms, but like any medication, they can also have side effects. Along with medications, psychotherapy is used as a treatment, either alone for milder illness or with antidepressants for more severe depression.

Many investigators have examined exercise as a treatment for mild to moderate depression. Usually, these training studies asked participants to exercise together three or four times a week. It is the regular physical activity, rather than being part of a training group, that lifts your spirits. We know that, because having people meet three times a week for an hour of stretching and muscle relaxation does not relieve depression. Also, in limited studies, an individualized program of home

---

TABLE 11.1   **Criteria for Depression**

Depression is indicated by two weeks of either a depressed mood or a markedly diminished interest or pleasure in your usual activities, plus at least one of the following:

- Weight loss when not dieting, or weight gain
- Insomnia or sleeping too much
- Restlessness or feeling slowed down
- Fatigue or lack of energy nearly every day
- Feelings of worthlessness or guilt
- Less ability to think or concentrate
- Recurrent thoughts of death or suicide

TABLE 11.2 **Beck Depression Inventory**

For each item, circle the number of the statement that best describes the way you feel right now. Add up the score for each of the 21 questions. The highest score for the 21 questions would be 63, and the lowest would be zero. The higher the score, the more severe your depression.

Score Range	Depression Level
1 to 10	Normal
11 to 16	Mild mood disturbance
17 to 20	Borderline clinical depression
21 to 30	Moderate depression
31 to 40	Severe depression
Over 40	Extreme depression

1. 0 I do not feel sad.
   1 I feel sad.
   2 I am sad all the time and I can't snap out of it.
   3 I am so sad or unhappy that I can't stand it.
2. 0 I am not particularly discouraged about the future.
   1 I feel discouraged about the future.
   2 I feel I have nothing to look forward to.
   3 I feel that the future is hopeless and that things cannot improve.
3. 0 I do not feel like a failure.
   1 I feel I have failed more than the average person.
   2 As I look back on my life, all I can see are a lot of failures.
   3 I feel I am a complete failure as a person.
4. 0 I get as much satisfaction out of things as I used to.
   1 I don't enjoy things the way I used to.
   2 I don't get real satisfaction out of anything anymore.
   3 I am dissatisfied or bored with everything.
5. 0 I don't feel particularly guilty.
   1 I feel guilty a good part of the time.

   2 I feel quite guilty most of the time.
   3 I feel guilty all of the time.
6. 0 I don't feel I am being punished.
   1 I feel I may be punished
   2 I expect to be punished.
   3 I feel I am being punished.
7. 0 I don't feel disappointed in myself.
   1 I am disappointed in myself.
   2 I am disgusted with myself.
   3 I hate myself worse than anybody else.
8. 0 I don't feel I am any worse than anybody else.
   1 I am critical of myself for my weaknesses and mistakes.
   2 I blame myself all the time for my faults.
   3 I blame myself for everything bad that happens.
9. 0 I don't have any thoughts of killing myself.
   1 I have thoughts of killing myself, but I would not carry them out.
   2 I would like to kill myself.
   3 I would kill myself if I had the chance.
10. 0 I don't cry any more than usual.
   1 I cry more now than I used to.
   2 I cry all the time.
   3 I used to be able to cry, but now I can't cry even though I want to.

TABLE 11.2   **Beck Depression Inventory** (*continued*)

11. 0 I am no more irritated by things than I ever am.
    1 I am slightly more irritated now than usual.
    2 I am quite annoyed or irritated a good deal of the time.
    3 I feel irritated all the time now.
12. 0 I have not lost interest in other people.
    1 I am less interested in other people than I used to be.
    2 I have lost most of my interest in other people.
    3 I have lost all of my interest in other people.
13. 0 I make decisions about as well as I ever could.
    1 I put off making decisions more than I used to.
    2 I have greater difficulty in making decisions than before.
    3 I can't make decisions at all anymore.
14. 0 I don't feel that I look any worse than I used to.
    1 I am worried that I am looking old or unattractive.
    2 I feel that there are permanent changes in my appearance that make me look unattractive.
    3 I believe that I look ugly.
15. 0 I can work about as well as before.
    1 It takes an extra effort to get started at doing something.
    2 I have to push myself very hard to do anything.
    3 I can't do any work at all.

16. 0 I can sleep as well as usual.
    1 I don't sleep as well as I used to.
    2 I wake up one or two hours earlier than usual and find it hard to get back to sleep.
    3 I wake up several hours earlier than I used to and cannot get back to sleep.
17. 0 I don't get more tired than usual.
    1 I get tired more easily than I used to.
    2 I get tired from doing almost anything.
    3 I am too tired to do anything.
18. 0 My appetite is no worse than usual.
    1 My appetite is not as good as it used to be.
    2 My appetite is much worse now.
    3 I have no appetite at all anymore.
19. 0 I haven't lost much weight, if any, lately.
    1 I have lost more than 5 pounds.
    2 I have lost more than 10 pounds.
    3 I have lost more than 15 pounds.
20. 0 I am no more worried about my health than usual.
    1 I am worried about physical problems such as aches and pains or upset stomach, or constipation.
    2 I am very worried about physical problems and it's hard to think of much else.
    3 I am so worried about my physical problems that I cannot think about anything else.
21. 0 I have not noticed any recent change in my interest in sex.
    1 I am less interested in sex than I used to be.
    2 I am much less interested in sex now.
    3 I have lost interest in sex completely.

exercise was shown to reduce depression just as well as working out with a group. Physical activity does not need to be vigorous for you to reap its psychological benefits. Just the opposite may be true, because some studies suggest that moderate physical activity will improve your mood more than high intensity exercise.

There are more than 35 studies of the effects of exercise on depression, and the combined results show that physical activity reverses mild to moderate depression as well as medications and psychotherapy. The more depressed you feel, the bigger its benefit. Even when you are not depressed, your mood will be better if you exercise. If you exercise regularly, your concentration is improved, and you sleep better. Studies consistently show that regular physical activity causes people to feel better and increases their sense of well-being.

In many ways, the psychological benefits of exercise are like those of an antidepressant. Like a medication, the psychological benefits of exercise begin weeks before you can measure any increase in your fitness level. The initial improvement is greatest if you are consistent with your training program. Just as with a drug, exercise is effective only if you take the medicine. Although the type and intensity of training do not seem to matter, the longer you maintain your program, the better the results. That is, three months of regular exercise will have a greater effect than six weeks of training. Similar to the effect of antidepressants, once you benefit from exercise, the improvement often persists, even though you may not be working out as consistently as during your initial training period.

Exercise has several psychological benefits that can reduce your feelings of depression. Regular physical activity increases your self-esteem and is a time-out or distraction from your daily stressors. Exercising with a partner or group also provides social support. Like antidepressant medications, a bout of exercise increases levels of dopamine and serotonin in your brain. The similarity in central nervous system effect may explain why physical activity and a medication can be combined effectively for treatment of depression.

Cindy's depression was mild or moderate in its severity. Although she often felt down and blue, she was still thinking clearly and finding joy in some activities. When asked about exercise, she was pessimistic about her ability to find the time, and she thought taking a pill to feel better would be easier. Cindy was caught in today's conundrum: too busy to exercise, but too busy not to.

St. John's Wort is a plant extract containing several chemicals. Studies show that it can improve symptoms of mild to moderate depression and anxiety. It occasionally causes side effects such as stomach upset, restlessness, and rashes.

SAD stands for *seasonal affective disorder*, which is a form of depression that occurs during the dark winter months. In addition to the usual findings of depression, people with SAD have a tendency to sleep too much, be socially withdrawn, crave sweet foods, and gain weight. (Like a bear hibernating for the winter.) Although SAD may be helped by exercise and antidepressant drugs, the primary treatment recommended by the American Medical Association and the American Psychiatric Association is light therapy: SAD's chemical imbalance, caused by long dark days, can be corrected by exposure to high-intensity light.

For all of us, memory is a poor guide to knowing how we spend our days. To help her discover when she might fit in physical activity, Cindy agreed to keep an activity log for one week, even though she felt it would be a waste of her already-limited time. She carried a small notebook and wrote down exactly what she did, as she did it—showering, getting dressed, driving, all the activities at work, shopping, folding clothes, even talking with her husband. She also kept track of her energy level, noting how she felt on a five-point scale (1 = fatigued, to 5 = energetic).

Before keeping the diary, Cindy thought the only way she could find time to exercise was by getting up 45 minutes earlier. With the log, she found that the morning was her most energized time of day, while after work and evenings were when she could best use the energy boost that can come from a bout of exercise. Cindy was surprised how much time she spent on some menial tasks. She saw that she often stopped at the store on the way home from work. Most of the time, her purchases were not needed urgently, but were items she had remembered while driving home—two bags of bark mulch, superglue to mend a broken vase, a single box of a certain cereal.

Cindy figured she could eliminate those trips by keeping a list of needed items and shopping only once or twice a week. That change freed up a little time, and she began taking her exercise clothes to work. Her gym bag on the back seat was a reminder that she needed to exercise, and she changed as she left the office. Three times a week, on her way home, she stopped to walk at a local track. She liked to listen to book audiotapes and be distracted from the day's events. Cindy was getting home at about the same time, already changed out of her work clothes and feeling more alert and refreshed. Her mood improved after only a couple of weeks of regular physical activity, and the increased energy that she felt made it easier to find the time for exercise.

Keeping an activity log can seem like a tedious task. However, its results are usually eye opening. Without a record, it is difficult to recall precisely how you spend your day, and what you do remember is usually not completely accurate.

Reducing Anxiety with Exercise

Jeffrey was a new patient, and before any conversation, I felt anxious just being in the same room with him. He was standing and pacing in the small exam room. Six months ago, he had made the decision to move to Oregon and assume a position with the Portland airport. At 36, Jeffrey described himself as high-strung. His work was demanding, and he was in the process of buying a house. Several years ago, he experienced panic attacks, and they were coming back. In addition, Jeffrey had a family history of high blood pressure. He often checked his blood pressure and was worried by a gradual increase in his readings. He took it as a sign to get help when he thought he heard his daughter's talking doll say, "We're going on medication," instead of, "We're going on vacation."

The operator paged with the message that a call from Florida was holding. Returning the page, the voice on the other end was our patient Alice, a 48-year-old nursing instructor who was attending a convention in Orlando. The previous night, she had experienced her first panic attack. She did not know what, if anything, triggered the spell, and her symptoms lasted less than five minutes. Alice was feeling fine now. She would not have called, except that she was worried about having another attack during the flight home.

Anxiety is an emotion everyone has experienced. It is a distressing feeling of apprehension and uneasiness. Being anxious causes changes in your thinking (fear, worry), bodily functions (rapid heart beat, sweating), and behavior (pacing, tapping the table), all of which only reinforce your feelings of distress. A little anxiety can be a good thing—like getting excited before an event or feeling up for a performance. Too much anxiety is not a good thing, and as shown in Figure 11.1, at a certain point, anxiety can impair your abilities.

The clinical anxiety syndromes include panic disorder, generalized anxiety disorder, phobias, and posttraumatic stress disorder.

The psychiatric problem *generalized anxiety disorder (GAD)* is much more than the normal anxiety that we all experience. It is an unprovoked chronic feeling of exaggerated worry and tension. Besides feeling anxious, people with GAD often have physical symptoms, such as trembling, twitching, headaches, diarrhea, sweating, or hot flashes. They may feel lightheaded, breathless, and as though they have a lump in the throat. Having this disorder means always anticipating disaster, and often worrying excessively about your health, money, family, and work.

Although sufferers know their anxiety level is more than they need, they cannot lessen their concerns. Just as with depression, anxious people do not have their condition by choice. They cannot control their feelings and will the anxiety away, without help. Successful treatment of GAD can include medication, psychotherapy, and relaxation techniques to control muscle tension.

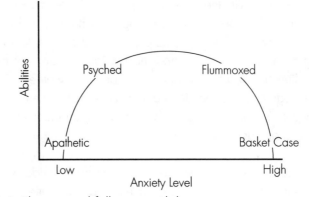

Figure 11.1 The rise and fall in your abilities as your anxiety increases

A panic attack is a discrete episode that occurs suddenly—your heart pounds, you may feel faint or dizzy, your hands may tremble, tingle, or feel numb, and you may have chest pain or a smothering sensation (Table 11.3). The feelings are terrifying, and you may think you are having a heart attack, stroke, or are about to die. Panic attacks can oc-

---

TABLE 11.3 **Panic Attacks**

A panic attack is an episode of intense fear or discomfort in which four (or more) of the following symptoms rapidly develop:

- Palpitations, pounding, or rapid heart beat
- Sweating
- Trembling or shaking
- Shortness of breath or smothering
- Choking sensation
- Chest pain
- Nausea or abdominal pain
- Feeling dizzy, unsteady, lightheaded, or faint
- Feelings of unreality or being detached from oneself
- Fear of losing control or going crazy
- Fear of dying
- Numbness or tingling sensations
- Chills or hot flushes

cur at any time without warning, even awakening you from sleep. They usually last a few minutes and occasionally persist for an hour or more.

You can have one panic attack and never have another. It is only with recurrent panic attacks that you qualify for having *panic disorder* (Table 11.4). Panic disorder affects almost 2 percent of us, and it is twice as common in women as in men. With this problem, you do not feel normal between panic attacks, and you have a persistent worry that another attack is right around the corner. Untreated, panic disorder can become disabling. Medications, a type of psychotherapy called cognitive-behavioral therapy, or a combination of the two can help most people with panic disorder.

Both a single bout and regular physical activity reduce your anxiety level. As with depression, physical activity achieves that effect in several ways. Being consistent with regular exercise increases your sense of personal control and mastery, which can counteract feelings of anxiety. A workout also may provide your mind with a distraction or diversion from stress. In addition, being in shape can lower your adrenaline levels. That is one of the reasons that your resting heart rate and blood pressure are lower after physical conditioning. When your adrenaline level is lower, even if you are anxious, you will have fewer physical changes (less rapid heart beat, less tremor, and less sweating). So, there will be fewer physical signals to reinforce your feelings of anxiety.

Although exercise reduces our anxiety levels, less research has been done concerning its use as a treatment for panic disorder or GAD. Regular physical activity appears helpful there, too. It can lower

Phobias are one of the anxiety syndromes. They are common and affect more than 1 in 10 people. A phobia is an intense, irrational fear of certain things or situations such as closed-in places, heights, or flying. Successful treatment usually involves a kind of psychotherapy called desensitization, in which patients are gradually exposed to what frightens them, until the fear begins to fade.

TABLE 11.4   **Panic Disorder**

Panic disorder is defined as recurrent panic attacks, persistent uncontrollable worry about panic attacks or their consequences (such as losing control, having a heart attack, or "going crazy"), and three (or more) of the following symptoms:

- Feeling restless or on edge
- Being easily fatigued
- Difficulty concentrating or your mind going blank
- Irritability or muscle tension
- Difficulty sleeping or restless unsatisfying sleep

As with depression, the recognition that anxiety disorders are common has helped reduce the stigma of this mental illness. Famous people who have suffered from an anxiety disorder include Isaac Asimov, Kim Basinger, Nicolas Cage, Earl Campbell, Johnny Depp, Sally Field, Aretha Franklin, Naomi Judd, John Madden, Alanis Morissette, Charles Schultz, Willard Scott, Barbra Streisand, and Oprah Winfrey.

Posttraumatic stress disorder (PTSD) can develop after you have been part of or witnessed a terrifying event. Those traumatic circumstances cause persistent frightening thoughts and feelings of emotional numbness. PTSD can occur at any age, including childhood, and it can be accompanied by depression, substance abuse, and anxiety. Antidepressants, anxiety-reducing medications, and psychotherapy are used in treating PTSD. Support from family and friends helps speed recovery.

anxiety levels and reduce the frequency of panic attacks. However, unlike with depression, where exercise alone may correct mild to moderate symptoms, regular physical activity is usually not enough to completely remedy the anxiety disorders. For those with GAD and panic disorder, exercise will help, but medications and psychotherapy will still be needed.

Jeffery was prescribed fluoxetine (Prozac). Although the SSRI (selective serotonin reuptake inhibitors) drugs are called antidepressants, they work equally well for anxiety. He also began a program of jogging three times a week during the noon hour. The exercise was a break for relaxation during the day, and the physical conditioning could benefit both his anxiety level and his blood pressure. Approximately five months later, when he had moved into his new home and things were better at work, the medication was tapered and stopped. Jeffery continues to exercise. He is no longer having panic attacks, and his blood pressure is normal.

Alice used alprazolam (Xanax), a short-acting benzodiazepine, to reduce anxiety on her flight home. She thought about what the panic attack might be telling her. She took it as the message, "You're closing in on 50, and it's time to reduce stress and take better care of your body." Among the lifestyle changes Alice made was beginning a program of swimming four times a week. She continues to travel to national meetings, and she has not had any further panic attacks.

Most people realize that aspects of their work, lifestyle, and own personality can cause stress. Too much stress can lead to fatigue, anxiety, depression, and physical illness. Regular physical activity is first on the list of ways to reduce chronic stress. Additional coping skills include rethinking an event's importance to put it in proper perspective, thinking positively ("I'm good enough, and people like me," [don't laugh, it can help]), and maintaining your sense of humor.

Exercise Addiction

J.T. works hard no matter what he does. He is a 47-year-old surgeon who sees a lot of patients, and when he is not in the operating room, J.T. is out exercising. He runs, pedals a stationary bike, and swims, all geared toward his competition in triathalons. These ultraendurance events combine a 2.4 mile swim, a 112 mile bike race, and a 26.2 mile marathon. J.T. first entered the Hawaiian Iron Man competition four years ago and has gone back each year, trying to improve his time. J.T. says that the event challenges him mentally and physically, and he likes to push his limits.

This year, J.T. was having problems. He felt fatigued. His back was "killing" him, especially when he ran. Even his patients remarked that he looked worn out. He prided himself on his lean appearance, but his weight had dropped another 10 pounds over the last two months. Although he knew about the importance of nutrition, he found he was usually too busy or too tired to eat properly.

Finally, the pain in his back became so intense that he ordered X rays of his spine. He was shocked to see that his back bones were thinned, with compression fractures of several vertebrae. Bone density studies confirmed he had osteoporosis. Rather than being a man of steel, his bones looked like those of an 80-year-old woman.

Exercise addiction is rare but real. For every person who overexercises, there are more than a hundred people who rarely exercise. Usually people who exercise regularly get along better at home and at work. To investigate how commonly exercise has an adverse impact, researchers surveyed the families of 1,500 members of a running club. The vast majority of families reported that they thought exercise was a good thing, and less than 5 percent reported that running was a cause of conflicts or problems.

Years ago, exercise physiologists thought that you could become addicted to exercise, much like you could be addicted to morphine. Vigorous exercise causes an increase in your levels of endorphins. The name *endorphin* comes from combining the two words *endogenous* (made in your body) and *morphine*, and these chemicals act on the same receptors as narcotics. Endorphin levels go up with most bouts of intense physical activity. Scientists used to think that endorphins accounted for a runner's high and explained why someone could get addicted to exercise.

Most intense workouts cause an increase in endorphin levels. One of the first exercise studies that we did showed that weight lifting causes your endorphin levels to go up, similar to the increase from running on a treadmill. Our bodies make endorphins whenever we exert ourselves, and the higher levels probably help us better tolerate discomfort. Imagine that you are one of your ancient ancestors and running away from a wooly mammoth. You want to be able to keep sprinting and ignore any physical pain, at least until you are safely back in your cave. That is where endorphins come in handy: they help block out physical discomfort. Despite higher endorphin levels, most people do not feel high after or get addicted to exercise

The causes of thinned bones are discussed in Chapter 3, pages 34–40. It is unusual for a man to have osteoporosis at J.T.'s age. However, his diet has been low in calcium most of his life. Even growing up, he never liked milk. Now, with his vigorous training, he was not getting enough total calories, protein, and minerals. When you work out as hard as J.T., your body needs extra calories to repair muscles, joints, and bones—tissues that you are using during your workouts. Without enough calories and building blocks, your tissues will weaken, and you will end up with an injury. The same process that can result in a stress fracture had weakened all of J.T.'s bones.

Exercise is considered an addiction when it prevents normal interactions at home or work. Just like any activity, people can be consumed with exercising: the more they exercise, the more they need to exercise. People with this problem may find it impossible to stop training, even though they become injured, and constantly strive to increase the intensity and length of their workouts.

How much is too much? Exercise addiction may be your problem if it pushes everything else in your life aside—family, friends, and other responsibilities. Table 11.5 lists additional questions to see whether you might be an exercise addict. Many times, exercise addiction is a clue to deeper problems, such as obsessive-compulsive disorder or depression, and professional help may be needed. The relationship between excessive exercise and eating disorders is discussed in Chapter 3, pages 47–49.

Concluding Remarks

Your head is healthiest when you exercise. Regular physical activity allows clearer thinking, reduces feeling of depression, lessens anxiety,

---

TABLE 11.5 **Are You an Exercise Addict?**

You might be an exercise addict if you answer yes to any of the following questions:
1. Your favorite video is *Buns of Steel*.
2. Your medicine cabinet contains ibuprofen, naprosyn, Bengay, and horse liniment.
3. Twelve pairs of athletic shoes line your closet floor.
4. The last time you missed exercising was during the Carter administration.
5. You think it's fun to be in pain.
6. Your dogs are named Nike and Adidas.
7. Your wedding was held at a road race, and Gatoraid and Powerbars were served at the reception.

---

and can correct insomnia. For those with mild to moderate depression, treatment with exercise is as effective as antidepressant medications. All types of regular exercise appear to provide these mental health benefits, and finding an activity that you enjoy may be more important than achieving a particular heart rate during training.

Chapter 12

Your Personal Exercise Prescription

It's 3 A.M. and you can't sleep. The television remote is lying near the phone on the mahogany nightstand. Grabbing the control, you push the "on" button. An attractive blond woman appears on the screen. She is explaining how a new device that twists your body one way and then the other while you pump up and down on the pedals, will make you lose inches and look years younger. The machine can perform this miracle with just four minutes of exercise each day! Several people are interviewed. They have been exercising on the twisting, pedaling thing for a few minutes, and they all say they like it. "It seems to tone," says one, whatever "tone" means. You remain skeptical. She is probably paid to say those words, and the people interviewed might be the only ones who like the device. Couldn't they select someone who has actually trained on the contraption?

You push a button on the remote, and the next channel advertises a peculiar item that claims to make your abdominal muscles tight, with a "ripped look." You see women and men showing their navels, laughing on the beach. There isn't an ounce of body fat on any of them. You think to yourself, "If I order the device, will I laugh on the beach with the beautiful people?" Again you push the channel selector. Channel 64 has yet another exercise gadget. This is something you sit on, pulling and pushing. Everyone looks happy riding it. But, they all look 20 years old, and you become concerned about your back and what that motion will do to it. You flip off the TV and try to go back to sleep. You are confused. Should you go for the abs and the beach, the twisting pedaling thing people like, or be happy with the riding unit? Well, tomorrow's another night.

We are bombarded with exercise infomercials every day. But the most dangerous time is late at night. Willpower is low, and the phone can gobble up your Visa or American Express number in seconds. When you feel compelled to buy exercise equipment past midnight, *don't do it!* Wait until morning. This way you will be fresh, your mind will be clear, and you can mull the purchase over and at least talk to someone else about it.

The First Rule of Fitness: Never buy any exercise device sold on television past midnight.

If you follow the First Rule of Fitness, you are much less likely to be one of the 88 percent of people who end up regretting their home exercise equipment purchase. It is not that all these devices are bad. Some are probably pretty good. But shop around. Before you invest any money, invest some time. The Second Rule of Fitness is, remember the First Rule of Fitness.

This chapter is designed to give you information about the different types of exercise you can do and how to train. We will explore definitions and the kind of exercise that will change your body, burn calories, improve your endurance, increase strength, and prevent and treat medical problems. After sifting through the following pages, you should be left with a pretty good idea of what you need to do and how to get there. So hold on to your hats and glasses, and get ready to start your engine.

Over 60 percent of home exercise equipment buyers state that they do not exercise regularly. Most people who purchase home fitness machines do so in the hope of starting an exercise program.

What Is Fitness?

Fitness means different things to different people. Who do you think is more fit, an elite endurance athlete who can run a 26 mile marathon in under 2.5 hours, or the weight lifter who can bench press 400 pounds? What about the person who can bend from his or her waist, legs straight, and can touch elbows to the floor? Would you ask the marathon runner to help you move a piano, or would you want the weight lifter to be on your team in a long-distance relay race? This is a little like comparing talented musicians who play different instruments. Can you compare a concert pianist with a violinist or a harpist? Which instrument sounds better? Who is the most accomplished?

Fitness is primarily a measure of your cardiovascular and musculo-skeletal system's response to physical activity. Being fit includes the following features: (1) aerobic capacity, (2) strength, (3) muscular endurance, and (4) joint flexibility. However, exercise also changes other body systems and functions. It can improve mood, lower your blood pressure, favorably change cholesterol levels, help control blood sugar levels, strengthen bones, and reduce the risk of heart disease and certain cancers. Although it is great to be fit, look trim, and appear more muscular, it is most important to translate fitness into health. Also, developing fitness is different from becoming an athlete. Athletes require not only fitness, but often need specific skills, coordination, and power. Although essential for most sports, these qualities are not necessary to gain 100 percent of the health benefits of exercise.

Just like a car burns gasoline to power its engine, your muscles burn organic fuels (mainly fats and carbohydrates) by combining them with oxygen to make energy for endurance activities. Your aerobic capacity, or maximal oxygen uptake (VO_2 max), is the most oxygen your muscles can use during endurance exercise. At rest you use approximately 3.5 mL of oxygen per kilogram of body weight to exist as a living human. This amount is conveniently referred to as 1 MET (metabolic equivalent). Oxygen uptake is often reported in numbers of METs. So if you are able to exercise 10 METs, your muscles can take up 35 mL oxygen/kg of body weight. In this example your body is sucking up 10 times the amount of oxygen you use at rest.

Elite runners can surpass 20 METs at peak exercise.

Strength is the capacity of your muscles to generate force for a brief period and does not rely on extra uptake of oxygen. The strength of specific muscle groups is often measured by the greatest ability to lift a particular weight once. This can be seen in Olympic weightlifting contests when a competitor lifts the heaviest weight possible. However, attempting a maximal lift is more likely to result in an injury. Tables in Appendix 1 can help you estimate the maximum amount of weight you can maximally lift, by hoisting a lesser weight as many times as you can.

Muscular endurance is a combination of aerobic ability and strength. It is a measure of your muscles' ability to repeat forceful movements without stopping. It is not the ability to lift the heaviest weight possible. For example, repeatedly lifting a weight that is about 40 to 60 percent of your maximal weight, or counting the number of push-ups you can do at one time is a measure of your muscular endurance.

Flexibility is your ability to stretch your muscles and tendons, providing greater joint mobility. Greater flexibility enables you to participate in activities with less risk of injury.

Table 12.1 lists the different types of fitness, their benefits, and how to achieve more of a good thing.

TABLE 12.1 **Types of Fitness and Their Benefits**

Fitness Type	What Is It?	Benefits	How to Improve
Aerobic capacity	Your ability to exercise over several minutes to hours at mild to moderate (not high) intensity. It requires oxygen to be absorbed by your lungs, then transferred to the bloodstream. Oxygen-rich blood is then pumped by your heart to your working muscles. Finally the oxygen is combined with fuel (mainly fats and carbohydrates), resulting in muscle energy.	Lowers blood pressure, improves blood sugar and cholesterol levels, burns fat, and helps prevent cardiovascular disease and cancer. Also, it can reduce depression and anxiety. Most benefits do not require more than a mild to moderate amount of training.	Maintain your exercise for a minimum of 15 minutes each workout. Although you achieve the greatest gain in aerobic capacity with three to four sessions at 30 minutes each week, daily exercise can improve your capacity and health, even more. Examples include walking, jogging, swimming, cycling, and dancing.
Strength	The ability of your muscles to create a burst of force, such as lifting, pushing, or pulling a weight. It does not require extra oxygen as does aerobic exercise. Strength is often measured by a person's maximal ability to lift a weight one time.	Strengthens bones, muscles, tendons; increases joint flexibility; lowers blood pressure; improves blood sugar and cholesterol levels; increases metabolic rate; and gives your body bulges in the right places. It creates a greater sense of confidence.	Warm up before training. Do not exercise the same major muscle groups two days in a row. Six to eight repetitions per set (one group of repetitions) for three to six sets. Stagger your workouts, for example, chest and back on one day, and legs and shoulders on another. Use correct form to avoid injury. Obtain enough rest between workouts. Eat foods high in carbohydrates and protein to replenish fuel stores and build muscle.
Muscular endurance	A combination of aerobics and strength training. It is the amount of exercise you can perform against moderate resistance, such as the number of push-ups you can do or the number of sprints you can run with short rest periods between runs.	Improves both aerobic fitness and strength. It can reduce body fat, lower blood pressure, improve cholesterol levels, and improve your ability to control blood sugar. It can improve joint flexibility.	Try 12 to 15 repetitions per set, using about 40 to 50 percent of the most you can lift. Don't train the same body parts two days in a row. It is best to exercise each muscle group in this manner every other day. Use active rest on nontraining days, and exercise aerobically.

TABLE 12.1 **Types of Fitness and Their Benefits** (*continued*)			
Fitness Type	**What Is It?**	**Benefits**	**How to Improve**
Flexibility	Your capacity to move your joints.	Reduces your risk of injury with exercise and daily activities, reduces the stress on muscles, tendons, and ligaments.	Stretch before and after your workout. Certain exercises, like yoga and Tai Chi, help promote flexibility.

What Do You Want Your Body to Be?

Mack and Cameron joined our exercise research study to become stronger and more fit. Mack, a 29-year-old phlebotomist (a person who draws blood in the laboratory), played football at a small Oregon college but had not exercised much in the past few years. His wife is pregnant with their first child, and for the first time he was concerned about his health. Although fit and muscular appearing, Mack had not exercised with weights, even during his college football days. His coach never believed in weight lifting for sport because he though it made athletes too inflexible and muscle-bound (contrary to his coach's opinion, proper weight lifting helps you become more flexible).

After just two weeks of training, Mack started adding weight to his frame. Sixteen weeks later, he weighed 16 pounds more than when he started, and testing showed that the added weight was all muscle. In fact, the body composition test revealed Mack to have gained 18 pounds of muscle and lost 2 pounds of fat. On the other hand, Cam is a 6 foot 1 inch, 32-year-old commercial real estate salesman who weighs 154 pounds. He is married with two small children. Cameron used to swim every day, but over the past few years, he did not have the time for exercise. Mack and Cam trained together. At the end of the study period, Cam had gained only 2 pounds of muscle. He was stronger and felt better, but he did not build as much muscle as fast as his training partner.

The experiences of Mack and Cameron illustrate how some people can respond differently to exercise. Both gained muscle, but Mack was able to gain at a faster pace. Had the training been an aerobic activity such as swimming, Cam may have become fitter faster.

There are two major types of benefical exercise: strength training (also called resistance exercise) and aerobics. Both types challenge your muscles in different ways. Likewise, muscles respond differently to each form of exertion. Resistance exercise, or weight lifting, stimulates our fast-twitch muscle fibers to contract with greater force, and given enough nutrients, our muscles become stronger and larger. Aerobic, or endurance, exercise forms more oxygen and fuel burning factories (mitochondrial oxidative enzymes in our muscle cells), especially in our slow-twitch muscles. This creates more dark muscle, but not the larger, bulkier white muscle. Because we are all different, some of us will attain higher levels of endurance at a much quicker pace, while others may become stronger faster. Some of us will continue to improve over months and even years, while others may improve for a while, then plateau. Also, there are nearly as many differences in our individual responses to each type of aerobic exercise (swimming versus jogging versus cycling) as there are between the different types of conditioning (aerobics versus strength training). However, there are few differences in the health benefits. Remember this: our bodies crave exercise and respond to physical activity with improved health. So select the exercise you enjoy.

> You need to eat about 2,500 extra calories of carbohydrate and protein to gain one pound of muscle.

My Body the Car

Think of your body as a vehicle. Some of us are like a fuel-efficient compact car, while others are made for strength, like a truck. However, most of us are in between, like a sports utility vehicle (SUV), while a few of us are quick and powerful like a dragster. Each one of these vehicles has unique properties. Athletes use the physical performance of these body types to compete in various sports, but we can all achieve some of those abilities with the right kind of exercise.

Distance runners, like the compact automobile, are not the fastest nor the most powerful vehicle, but they have the most endurance. On the other hand the SUV, like some hockey players or football linebackers are rugged, participate well in most sports, and combine strength and endurance. The truck is more like the large, bulky football lineman; it is very strong and able to pull and lift heavy loads, but it doesn't have the fuel efficiency of a compact car or SUV and is slower moving. The dragster, like the 100 meter sprinter or Olympic weight lifter, is fast, quick, and powerful for brief periods. It uses a lot of fuel, but does not necessarily have a lot of endurance.

Customizing Your Body

The engine you are about to construct consists of your muscles. The fuel pump is your heart and blood vessels. By choosing aerobic exercises, you train your heart and muscles to have greater endurance. When you train your cardiovascular system and muscles to become more like an SUV, you select a combination of aerobics and strength training. Truck training usually calls for heavy weight lifting, while dragster exercises rely on specific types of burst training, performing specialized exercises with jumping and speed drills, that is more often used for competitive athletics.

The type of exercise you choose depends on the type of vehicle you want to make. Do you want to be a fuel-efficient, high-endurance compact, or a powerful 16-wheeler, or an SUV with the ability to handle all terrain? Maybe you want to develop your own concept body and choose a little from each model? You have some choices to make.

The Engine

The muscles of the human body are composed primarily of two fiber types: a slow-twitch group, best used for endurance, and a fast-twitch type, which is best for strength and speed. Slow-twitch fibers desire oxygen and use fat and sugar as fuel. They are rich in microscopic energy factories called mitochondria, where oxygen combines with your body's fuel (fat and sugar) to create energy for muscle movement.

Our fat stores are our body's major fuel tank. Your slow-twitch fibers want fat and use it just like a candle burning wax. A candle radiates light at a low intensity, but it lasts for a very long time. Fats cannot be used for short bursts of intense exercise.

The fast-twitch speed and strength fibers love carbohydrates during bursts of activity and do not need a large supply of oxygen . . . at least not right away. Carbohydrates are your high-octane fuel, creating a flame more like a blow torch instead of a candle. High-intensity

Training fuels: Your muscles use carbohydrates (sugars and starches) and fats (oils and milk fats, etc.) as fuels for exercise. Carbohydrates are high-performance gas, necessary for speed and power, and are quickly consumed. Fats are low-performance fuels, used mainly for lower-intensity exercise such as walking and slow jogging. As you increase the intensity of exertion, more carbohydrates are burned. The *additives* (vitamins and minerals) are contained in the foods you eat and help convert fuel into energy.

Do you have the ability to be a champion marathoner? You better have been born with a lot of slow-twitch fibers in your legs.

exercise will take more oxygen later, right after the exercise. Blow-torches burn hot and bright, but the effect does not last very long. You build up an oxygen debt, which must be repaid with heavy breathing at the end of your intense activity.

Training affects your muscle fibers. When you begin a jogging program, the slow-twitch fibers increase their capacity to take up oxygen. If you begin burst activities such as weight training or sprinting, these fibers will develop more fast-twitch properties. No matter what your fiber types, you might not ever be able to win the Olympic marathon, be competitive in a local weight-lifting contest, or out run the 13-year-old neighbor in the 50 yard dash. But, you can improve your aerobic abilities and strength by exercising. Importantly, your health can be as great as that of an Olympic champion.

Should you train for the 100 meter dash? You will need an abundance of fast-twitch fibers in your legs.

Aerobic Training

Aerobic exercise, also called endurance or cardiorespiratory conditioning, requires you to tap into the type of energy used for continuous, nonstop exertion that lasts more than a few minutes. To supply your body with energy during aerobic exercise, you first breathe oxygen into your lungs. This oxygen is filtered into your bloodstream and attaches to red blood cells. The oxygen-rich blood is distributed to exercising muscles by your fuel pump, the heart. Finally, oxygen enters the cells of your exercising muscles, is transported into the mitochondria, and combines with fat and sugar to create energy. As you get in shape, muscles improve their ability to take up oxygen and use fat and sugar fuels. It takes several weeks to notice improvements when you change your muscle cells' abilities to produce more energy during exercise.

Aerobic exercise causes your body's engine (your muscles) to become like a fuel-efficient compact car. You are able to travel great distances, whether your training is walking, swimming, jogging, cycling, or other similar activity.

Specificity of Training

Although the health benefits are similar for all aerobic activities, one type of endurance training does not automatically transfer to another type of aerobic exertion. For example swimming every day will not necessarily make you a better jogger. Those who swim are training their muscles to become more fit for a swimming motion, while those who jog are becoming fitter joggers. Also, training your legs by running will not improve the aerobic capacity of your arms. Some exercises have a little more overlap, but not as much as you might think. This phenomenon is referred to as the specificity of training. That is why triathalons are so difficult. You need to specifically train for three different aerobic events: swimming, cycling, and long-distance running. Such athletes need the time and energy to train for three people.

Sally is a good friend. When she was in college at the University of Oregon, Sally spent the summer at her parents' home in Bethesda, Maryland. Her soon-to-be husband Dave was traveling in Europe. While awaiting his return, Sally, who always worked out, became even more diligent in her exercise routine. Running as much as 10 miles each day, in addition to biking and occasional laps in the local pool, she awaited the return of her true love by burning up the road with long runs and miles of cycling. Shortly after returning to Oregon, she recounted her summer's exercise routine. "I can't believe how fit I am," she exclaimed. "I am la machine." Dr. Goldberg tried to explain that her legs may have been in great aerobic shape, but her arms were probably no more fit than when she left Oregon in early June. Sally argued that her heart and lungs were in incredible shape. "No way, I literally can't get tired," she laughed. To put her to the test, Dr. Goldberg gave her some boxing gloves for a friendly sparring session. He promised not to punch back; he would just try to avoid her punches. Sally thought this would be great. Having grown up with three older brothers, she had years of experience and was ready to go. Slipping the gloves on, she thought the debate would be answered with her ability to continue punching for a very long while without fatiguing. Swinging as hard as she could, Sally punched at her moving target, but her gloves mainly flailed at the air. In a little more than a minute, her blows became weaker and weaker. Within three minutes, Sally was bent over, gasping for breath, and unable to continue. La machine was worn out.

Twenty years later and still "madly in love with Dave," Sally, now a nurse and mother of three, continues to exercise regularly and participates in various athletic events from fun runs to marathons. She does push-ups three days each week to give her upper body some exercise, too. A boxing rematch has not been scheduled.

Strength Training

The basic principle of strength training is to make muscles work against resistance. Resistance is usually in the form of weights, but can include bands, springs, compressed air, or our body weight, you name it. When you perform a resistance exercise such as a pull-up, your biceps muscle shortens as your elbow bends. This is called an isotonic contraction. Isotonic means that that there is the same resistance or tension throughout the movement. However, when there is so much resistance that you can't budge the grand piano or are unable to open a jar of pickles, it is an isometric exercise. The muscle tension builds, but the muscle doesn't shorten or lengthen. Isometric exercise will still strengthen the muscle, but it is not a very effective training method because of limited joint movement. Many of us feel like isometric people from time to time, exerting as hard as we can but seemingly not getting anywhere.

We have been advocates of pumping iron and other types of resistance exercise for years, before it became popular with the general public. In fact, our first major exercise study, published in the *Journal of the American Medical Association,* involved men and women who entered into a weight-lifting program and successfully reduced their cholesterol and triglyceride levels.

Despite that study and the many other research projects showing the benefits of resistance exercise, many misconceptions remain. These include the belief that strength training will create an inflexible and muscle-bound body and make you lose your coordination. Strength training actually improves flexibility and coordination. Professional, Olympic, college, and high school trainers and coaches understand this today, and resistance exercise is used for all sports, including swimming, tennis, and golf. But you do not need to lift heavy weights and develop bulging biceps to benefit. You can reshape your body, stoke your metabolic furnace to burn more calories, and gain all the health benefits from pumping iron without the need to lift heavy weights.

As we push and pull against resistance, our muscles respond to the challenge and become stronger. There are two ways this occurs. First your strength increases by coordinating more muscle fibers to contract together. This effect occurs after just a few training sessions, before there is any change in muscle size. Unlike aerobic training, you can notice an increase in strength within one to two weeks. A second and much more gradual effect occurs as your muscle fibers become larger and stronger.

Iso means *same* and *metric* means *length.* So the term *isometric* literally means *same length.* This occurs when muscle movement is attempted and no movement can take place because there is too much resistance. *Isotonic* means *same resistance* (*same tone*). Isotonic contractions occur when there is similar resistance present during the muscle movement, such as lifting a weight. During an isotonic exercise the muscle changes its length and contracts.

Weight lifting strengthens tendons and ligaments, increases bone density, and builds muscle. More muscle means a higher metabolic rate and more fat-burning power.

Although there are numerous strength-training programs, each is based on three major types of strength training, and each of the three produces distinct results. Contrary to what some people believe, there is no "best" strength training program. We call the three major types of strength gaining programs (see Table 12.5), Sport Utility Vehicle (SUV), Truck, and Dragster training.

SUV Training

SUV conditioning uses light to moderate weight, equal to about half the maximal weight you can lift just once. Twelve to 15 repetitions are performed in each set of repetitions, without stopping. The rest period between each set of exercises is brief and should be no more than 15 to 30 seconds. This type of conditioning builds strength, coordination, and muscular endurance. It helps teach your nerves and muscles to work together and perform each lift efficiently. It is the only type of weight lifting that builds aerobic capacity along with strength. This training is preferred by many exercise scientists because it promotes health without creating more severe stress on your joints, tendons, and ligaments as other heavier and more "explosive" types of strength training may do.

Truck Training

Trucks are designed to lift heavy cargo, but they are not fuel efficient and do not require extreme quickness or nimble movements. Truck training builds the greatest increases in strength by using heavier weights (about 75 percent or more of a person's maximum lift) and fewer repetitions (typically four to eight per set) than SUV training. Because of the greater resistance to muscular movement, the muscles undergo a high degree of stress and respond by becoming larger. Rest periods are longer and take from two to four minutes before lifting again. Although the fastest strength gains are achieved with this style of weight training, little or no aerobic fitness improvements occur, and constant use of heavy weights increases your chance of injury.

Dragster Training

Dragsters are explosive vehicles that combine speed and strength. Training like a dragster means explosive training, such as repeated jumps and skips, and using throwing movements when lifting weights. Although these exercises can enhance an athlete's physical performance, there is little or no research about the health benefits of this style of training. In addition, dragster training is more likely to cause an injury. We do not recommend dragster training for those who are not engaged in competitive athletics.

When you use resistance training, your muscles need about 48 hours to repair. Do not strength train the same muscle group two days in a row.

Exercise for the Ages

Lou is a retired dentist and former dean of the state's dental school. He is nearly 74 years old and has been married for 50 years. His body build is more like that of a muscular 40-year-old. He walks with a spring in his step and has a perpetual smile on his face. Lou's exercise is low tech. He walks four miles every other day and performs his brand of strength training on alternate days. No fancy equipment in his home gym, the resistance exercise Lou chooses includes using an old-fashioned elastic band to pull across his chest and two 20 pound dumbbells. All of this is complemented with hours of shoveling, planting, and pruning on his 1.5 acre backyard. Even as the elder patriarch of a large family, he still remains the champion arm wrestler. "You can maintain your health and do what you want to do, no matter what age you are," said Lou during his last physical examination. "If you don't use it, you lose it."

Lou shows us that we can continue to exercise and be very fit as we grow older. He just seems to keep going and going and going. Although he is an uncommon individual, his fitness story is not unique. In a study of athletes of all ages, older athletes had the same healthy metabolic profile as young athletes. This was much superior, both to older and younger inactive people. Fitness is as close to Ponce de Leon's fountain of youth as we can get.

If you live long enough, you will have to face old age.—H. Turtledove (exercising 77-year-old patient)

Exercise Equipment

Just a few years ago, the extent of home exercise equipment included an exercycle, some free weights, and a jump rope. Not a lot of variety. Some of these items were fine, but they were pretty low tech and you

In a survey of more than 8,000 readers who had home exercise machines, motorized treadmills were the "best bet" in home exercise equipment, as judged by Consumer Reports (February, 1999). While 53 percent continued to use motorized treadmills regularly, only 27 percent continued to use the nonmotorized form.

had to be really dedicated to use them consistently. We remember the first inexpensive home exercycles of the 1970s. After just one week, every time you dialed up the tension, you would nearly pass out from the toxic fumes of the burning rubber resistance wheel. It took about 20 minutes before the wheel could be touched without sustaining third-degree burns.

Today you can equip your home nearly as well as a commercial gym. This equipment can be general, or quite specialized. Some machines are used for aerobic conditioning, some are designed for strength training, and others tend to stimulate both strength and endurance. Table 12.2 describes the major types of exercise equipment you can find in gyms and purchase for home use. Don't even think about purchasing these machines unless you are committed to using them. Even the best equipment is worthless if it only gathers dust in your garage.

TABLE 12.2   **The Lowdown on Common Training Equipment**

Equipment	What It Does	What You Want
Treadmill Comes in various equipment grades: Economy grade supports up to 200 pounds ($800–$1,500) and is best for walking and light jogging; mid-priced supports up to 230 pounds ($1,800–$2,500) for walking and light jogging; premium treadmills ($2,600–$3,500) can support 250 pound joggers; commercial treadmills for fitness and testing centers cost $4,000–$7,500 or more.	Excellent for aerobic training. Builds aerobic fitness and burns as many or more calories than any other exercise machine, including cross country skiers and combination upper and lower extremity exercisers. It has a much softer surface than concrete or asphalt, making it less stressful on the ankles, knees, and hips.	Comes in more expensive motorized forms and nonmotorized models. Nonmotorized belts often do not glide smoothly. Should have guard rails on the side and at the front of the treadmill to use for balance, and a nonskid surface. Treadmill deck and belt should be rated for about 6,000 miles. Some models have reversible belts that double the life of the belt. For motorized, ask for a 2 HP motor. Try the treadmill before buying and have a 30 day minimum return policy with a 1 or 2 year warranty.

TABLE 12.2   **The Lowdown on Common Training Equipment** (continued)

Equipment	What It Does	What You Want
Exercycle Usual cost for a new cycle is between $250 and $1,400 for home models.	Very good aerobic device. Burns about 10 percent fewer calories than a treadmill. Low impact with less stress on the joints, especially useful for those who are 30 or more pounds overweight or have arthritis. Preferred exercise for those who have reduced blood flow to their legs. Recumbent cycles are chairlike and less stressful on your lower back.	Cheaper models do not last long and can lose their tension over time. Make sure the seat is comfortable and that it is adjusted to the proper height (when the pedal is at its lowest point, your knee is almost straight). Make sure the cycle is guaranteed for 1 year. The pedaling should be smooth.
Stair Climber Basic models start at $600. More elaborate climbers cost $2,000–$2,500.	Can be an excellent low-impact aerobic device when used correctly. The main problem is trying to exercise at a level that is too high, while supporting some weight on the side rails. Nonmotorized home models have difficult-to-adjust tension to accommodate different weights and fitness levels.	Exercise stroke should be smooth. You should perform a complete exercise session to determine the machine's stability and performance. Be sure that the stepper can be changed to different intensity levels. Inexpensive home models are often not adequate for long-term training.
Elliptical Machine Basic models start at $500; commercial grade is about $3,500.	Can provide excellent, low impact conditioning for your legs. Some machines have arm levers you can use for your upper extremities. These aerobic machines are really extensions of bicycle pedals on long boards, making your stride move in an elliptical motion. Good machines feel like you are gliding, with little impact. Home model strides may be shorter and provide less range of motion.	Nonskid surface and the ability to increase the level of difficulty. Make sure the stride length feels long enough and that the machine can support your weight. Use a gym's machine first, before purchasing. Commercial machines often accommodate up to 350 pounds. Many home fitness machines are flimsy and have short strokes, which make it more difficult to gain aerobic benefits.

TABLE 12.2   **The Lowdown on Common Training Equipment** (*continued*)

Equipment	What It Does	What You Want
Rower Basic models start at $600; commercial grade is about $2,000.	Rowing machines offer the benefit of an all-over workout with little impact on the joints. Excellent back and upper and lower extremity aerobic, strength and flexibility conditioning. Also strengthens your upper back. Does not typically burn as many calories as a treadmill. Some do not increase workload unless you row faster. Not the exercise of choice if you have low back pain or low back problems.	The stroke must be smooth and have a full range of motion, with a comfortable sliding seat. A word of caution: rowing can place stress on the lower back. A large variation in models. Some are excellent, but not compact. Some are compact, but do not provide higher-intensity workouts.
Cross Country Skier Basic models begin at $250, but more substantial skiers begin at about $600.	Uses both upper and lower extremities for total body aerobic conditioning. Does not burn as many calories as a motorized treadmill because of lower overall exercise intensity.	Some people have trouble coordinating their arms and legs with this exerciser. Use a skier that will increase its training intensity, either by elevating the skiing platform or increasing the tension.
Rider Usually start at $300.	Exercises the arms, legs, and upper back, with low impact. Some models have the ability to increase work by altering the tension. These are preferred. Many models appear to be designed for those with lower aerobic fitness, so can be helpful for those who are older and less fit. Calorie burning may be low.	Make sure you can increase the exercise workload. Be careful if you have low back discomfort or a history of low back pain. In one survey, most people who purchased riders (78%) did not continue regular use.
Home Gym Basic models begin at $500–$600.	Many different models to choose from. Will build strength and muscular endurance. Some machines are easier than others for changing exercises. Machines that allow for two-way resistance (resistance when you lift and when you return the bar or handles) are the best.	Some machines have a very jerky motion. You want the movement to be smooth. Don't be impressed by videos of someone who has used the machine. Make sure you try the machine and that it fits your body and is comfortable to use. Some are large and inconvenient.

Training Suggestions

Building the Compact Car

Your aerobic fitness, or endurance capacity, improves slowly over weeks, so do not think your gains will miraculously appear within a few days after starting. If you are just beginning, easy does it. Remember that you are in this for the long haul. Regular exercise is just like a savings account, but it will pay dividends in health benefits.

Only 25 percent of home exercise machines are used long-term.

Your exercise prescription has several ingredients, as shown in Table 12.3.

Mode

You have a number of ways to train aerobically, but all share in the continuous use of larger muscle groups. After several weeks, your heart works more efficiently, pumping more blood with each beat, and your muscles are able to use more oxygen from the blood, creating greater endurance capacity. Whether you choose walking, jogging, swimming, various exercise machines, skating, or cycling, the health benefits are very similar.

Intensity

Intensity is the amount of effort you expend during the exercise, or how hard you are working. Because each of us has a different capacity, you, not the exercise, determine your training intensity. For example, jogging three miles at a 10 minute per mile pace may be very difficult for some of us, while for others, it doesn't feel like much exertion at all.

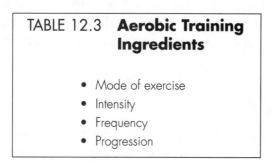

TABLE 12.3 **Aerobic Training Ingredients**

- Mode of exercise
- Intensity
- Frequency
- Progression

To gain endurance, there are four ways to find out how intense your aerobic training should be. One involves your measured heart rate during an exercise test, another is a formula, the third is related to your breathing and ability to talk during the activity, and the fourth is how you feel as you train. The maximal exercise test is often performed by physicians and exercise technicians in a laboratory, while you walk and run on a motorized treadmill, or pedal a stationary cycle. During this test, your maximal heart rate is measured with sophisticated heart monitoring devices (usually an electrocardiogram). Measuring your maximal heart rate is more accurate than predicting it from the formula: 220 − your age = your maximal heart rate. The predicted maximal heart rate for a 50-year-old man or woman would be approximately 170 beats per minute. His training heart rate should be between 65 and 85 percent of the maximum, or between 110 and 145 beats per minute. If you are just beginning to exercise, your training heart rate should be at the low end of the range. Although not necessary for health, as you become more fit, you can increase the training intensity up to 85 percent of your maximal heart, if you wish to boost your aerobic fitness to its highest level.

Another way to estimate exercise intensity is based on your breathing and ability to talk. As you train, you should be able to talk comfortably in short sentences. However, you should not have enough breath to sing. If you are able to say only a few words between gasps, you are exercising too intensely. The last method of training intensity is based on how you feel. If you are the more sensing type, try the Borg perceived exertion scale. It is easiest to use the 10-point scale (Table 12.4). Your rating should indicate your overall feeling, not whether you have a pain in your leg and want to stop exercising.

When you begin your program, exercise at level 2. If you were to check your heart rate, it would be at about 65 to 70 percent of your maximum. Many of the benefits of regular aerobic exercise, including an increase in fitness, lower blood pressure, less chance of diabetes, and a longer life, can be achieved with this level of exertion. As you continue training, you can move your intensity to a 3 or 4 to raise your aerobic fitness.

Duration

How long should each exercise session last? In the words of the ancient Chinese proverb (which we have modified), a journey of 1,000 miles

Finding your exercise heart rate: There are two methods to determine your exercise heart rate. One way is to purchase a heart rate monitor or use aerobic equipment with built-in heart rate sensors. Also, you can check your heart rate the old fashioned way, using a finger, and save a lot of money. Immediately after exercise or while on the training device (if possible), feel your pulse with your index finger of the opposite hand at the wrist, just above the base of your thumb. Look at your watch and count the beats for 10 seconds, then multiply by 6. This is a close estimate of your exercise heart rate.

TABLE 12.4 **Modified Borg Exertion Scale**

Number	Verbal Response
0	Nothing
0.5	Very, very weak
1	Very weak
2	Weak
3	Moderate
4	Somewhat strong
5	Strong
6	Strong plus
7	Very strong
8	Really, really strong
9	I can only do this a few more seconds
10	Okay, stop! I give up.

Modified from Borg GA, Med Sci Sports Exerc 14:377–387.

begins with the first step. Similarly, your exercise program can begin with as little as 10 minutes of activity. In fact, we often tell patients to start walking away from their home, walk for 5 minutes, then turn around and come back. They have exercised 10 minutes and it was painless. Each session, add 30 seconds to the journey away from home (1 minute overall), and within a few weeks, you will be exercising for 30 minutes. *Then you can say you "walk the walk."*

Most research indicates that 30 minutes is a standard training period, but you don't have to exercise for half an hour all at one time. Ten minutes, three times during the day is effective, too. This can be helpful for people with busy schedules who are just trying to fit some activity into their day.

Frequency

Frequency refers to the number of times you exercise each week. Although there is no magic number, research shows that the frequency needed to achieve the benefits of exercise is approximately three times per week. With only three sessions per week, make sure you spread your workout over the week and do not go more than 72 hours (preferably not more than 48 hours) without exercising. Being a weekend warrior is not enough. In fact, without regular exercise, you are more likely to become injured.

For those who are just starting out, three sessions per week is sufficient. After six weeks, your muscles and tendons are ready for you to boost your exercise frequency to four or more times each week. If you have a condition such as diabetes or if you are trying to lose excess body fat, it is better to exercise every day, even if it is only 10 to 15 minutes.

Regular aerobic training will improve your endurance by a whopping 25 percent within eight weeks! Try boosting your bank account by 25 percent in two months!

Progression

As you continue to train, your capacity to exercise steadily increases, enabling you to add on more work without it seeming like more. The initial improvement stage lasts about six to eight weeks. During this time, the enzyme levels in your muscles' mitochondria (your energy factories) increase, and your heart is able to pump more blood to your muscles. Also, we mention progression as a reminder to not exercise so hard or long that you cause an injury. To improve even more, you can increase your exercise intensity, duration, or frequency, or all three. But no matter what you decide to do, always build slowly.

Build up to 30 minutes of exercise, three times each week, and continue this level for about two months before increasing the amount of time or exercise intensity. Then, gradually increase the amount of exercise every four weeks, either by intensity (add 5 percent to your training heart rate each month until you achieve a heart rate between 80 and 85 percent of maximum), frequency (add one day each week, until you are exercising five to seven days each week), or add 5 to 10 minutes each exercise session, until you are exercising about 45 minutes to 1 hour each session.

Everything else being equal, higher-intensity exercise is more likely to increase your aerobic fitness more than exercising longer or more frequently. Also, high-intensity aerobics are more likely to rearrange your cholesterol levels. However, changing the intensity of your training is a little different than extending the time you train or scheduling more training periods. When you boost your exercise intensity from 65 percent to 80 percent of your maximal heart rate, it is a big jump in

For most benefits of aerobic exercise, including lowering blood pressure, burning fat, and giving you a psychological boost, lower-intensity exercise is as beneficial as more vigorous training.

your level of perceived exertion. So it becomes more difficult to keep up the pace for the same period of time.

Building Stronger Muscles

Although, there is no "best" strength-training program, the three basic types are Sports Utility Vehicle, Truck, and Dragster training. The specifics of each type of strength conditioning are listed in Table 12.5. We recommend SUV training for everyone. Truck training is for those who need more strength for athletics or a specific job, and the Dragster is mainly for competitive athletes. There are more injuries with Truck and Dragster training.

Remember, there is no need for the appearance of "ripped" abdominal muscles and bulging biceps to gain the health benefits of strength training. Before you rush to join a gym or purchase your own weights, you might want to try the home strength-training assessment in Table 12.6 to see where you are right now. By doing this assessment, you can keep a record of your progress over the next few months. If

TABLE 12.5 **Three Major Types of Strength Training**

Features	Sport Utility	Truck	Dragster
Training weight	Moderate (about 50% of your maximum lift)	Heavy (70–85% of your maximum lift)	Moderately heavy (50–70% of your maximum lift)
Repetitions/set	12–15	4–8	4–10
Number of sets in each workout	3–4	6–8	Varies 2–6
Rest intervals between sets	15–30 seconds	2–4 minutes	1–2 minutes
Major physical benefits	Muscular endurance++* Muscle blood flow+ Strength+ Muscle size+ Aerobic fitness+	Strength++ Muscle size++ Power+	Explosive power++ Speed and quickness++ Strength+

*+, an increase; ++, a very high increase.

TABLE 12.6   **Quick Home Strength Assessment**

Arms and Chest

Do as many push-ups as you can. Make sure you keep your back straight. Your chest should just touch the floor. Women should perform a modified push-up with knees resting on the floor.

- High fitness = 25 or more
- Moderately high = 20–24
- Average = 15–19
- Below Average = 10–14
- Way below average = 5–9
- Nowhere to go but up = 0–4

Torso

Lying on your back, place your arms behind your neck, in the sit-up position. Now hold a 45 degree angle for as long as you can, without pulling on your neck.

- High level = 40 or more seconds
- Moderately high = 30–39 seconds
- Average = 20–29 seconds
- Below average = 15–19 seconds
- Way below average = 10–14 seconds
- Nowhere to go but up = 0–9 seconds

Legs

The wall sit exercise can be performed by leaning against a wall; bend your legs so that your knees are at a 90 degree angle. Hold this position as long as you can.

- High = 90 seconds
- Moderately High = 80–89 seconds
- Average = 60–79 seconds
- Below Average = 40–59 seconds
- Nowhere to go but up = 39 seconds or less

---

you want to know how strong you are, there is no need to perform a maximum lift to see how much you can lift just once. By using a weight you can lift maximally 2 to 10 times, you can calculate your 1-RM (one-repetition maximum) (see Appendix 1). The terms used in strength training are defined in Table 12.7.

TABLE 12.7 **Strength Training Definitions: Talking the Talk**

1-RM: The maximum weight a person can lift when performing a particular exercise is termed a one-repetition maximum, or 1-RM.

Circuit training: Builds muscular endurance and is a form of "Sports Utility" training. This form of strength training typically uses a variety of exercises with lower weights (about 40–60% of your 1-RM) and more repetitions (12–15 per set). You quickly move from one exercise to the next with only a few seconds of rest, often alternating upper body and lower body exercises.

Cycling: This has nothing to do with bicycles. It means, changing your workout program every one or two months. This may involve changing the amount of weight, the number of repetitions, or both. This helps challenge the muscles for continued improvement.

Muscular hypertrophy: Muscle tissue is made of individual muscle fibers. When enough calories and protein are available for muscle growth, strength training causes an increase in the size of fibers (hypertrophy).

Periodization: This technique rotates different types of strength-training programs. Each type lasts a few weeks to months, depending on the needs or desires of the exerciser. This type of training is thought to result in greater gains with fewer injuries.

Power: This is a combination of strength and speed. You can increase your power by lifting the weight faster or adding more weight.

Pyramid sets: Each set of exercises begins with a lighter weight and more repetitions. With the next few sets, more weight is added with fewer repetitions for each set.

Repetitions (reps): This is the number of times a particular weight is lifted during a set.

Set: A group of repetitions. For example, when a person performs a bench press 10 times, this is *one set* of *10 repetitions* (reps).

Strength: The muscle's ability to produce force. Strength can be measured by finding the maximum weight you can lift for a certain exercise. However, since lifting at 1-RM can be dangerous, it is better to choose a lower weight and measure the number of repetitions.

No matter whether you are a beginner or a long-time exerciser, you want to get the most out of your training, without injury. To do this you need to work slowly over the first several weeks while your muscles are learning to overcome the resistance to movement, and the tendons are being stressed in new and different ways. Above all, rest is critical! This is true especially in the early training stages. When you are not exercising, your muscles refuel and undergo repair from the trauma of training. This allows them to become bigger and stronger, while the tendons that attach your muscles to bone become more resilient and create firmer attachments. Too much work too fast leads to injury.

Although there are different types of training and different weight lifting machines, there are a few basic rules you should follow, listed in Table 12.8.

TABLE 12.8   **Basic Strength-Training Rules**

- Warm up with stretching and at least 5 minutes of aerobic exercise (see stretching examples on pages 246–252) before you lift.
- Work the larger muscle groups (chest, back, thighs) first, before training your smaller muscles (triceps, biceps, calves)
- Rest the muscle groups you trained for at least 24 hours after lifting (you can do aerobics, but not strength training)
- Use correct form (cheating leads to injury)
- Aim for a weight you can lift between 8 and 15 times
- Gradually increase the weight you lift by 5 percent

Your Program

Breathing techniques are an important part of weight lifting and reduce the stress on your heart and cardiovascular system. Do not hold your breath while you lift weights. Inhale through your nose just prior to exertion. Then exhale through gently pursed lips as you lift the weight.

Let us make a suggestion. If you are a beginning weight lifter, start with the eight exercises listed in Table 12.9 to begin your strength-training routine. These exercises will strengthen all your major muscle groups and prepare you for other lifts down the road. Remember, when you first select a weight, choose one you are able to lift between 8 to 15 times. On your first day of strength-training, complete only one set of each exercise. On the second day, two days later, perform two sets of each exercise. Then on the third day, perform three sets. After that, every time you exercise perform three sets for each exercise. When you can lift a weight 15 times for each of three sets, increase the weight by approximately 5 percent.

Training Examples

The following workout examples can be used for basic strength conditioning. There are many other strength-training workouts you can use, but these can get you on the right track. Using a personal trainer at a local gym can be very worthwhile. Select one who has been certified by national organizations such as the American College of Sports Medicine, American Federation of Weightlifting, and the American Council on Exercise.

TABLE 12.9 **The Muscle-Building Exercises That Work**

1. Bench Press (Figures 12.1 & 12.2)

Muscles strengthened: Chest, back of the arms, front of the shoulders, and upper back.

Position: Lie with your back and head flat on the bench, legs to the side and feet on the floor.

Grip: Overhand with thumbs wrapped around the bar.

Motion: The bar should lightly touch the chest, just above the nipple line, for a count of "one," then lift slowly without jerking.

Breathing: Inhale as you lower the weight, exhale as you raise the bar.

2. Leg Press or Back Squat (Figure 12.3)

Leg Press

Muscles strengthened: Front of thighs, back of thighs, and hips.

Position: Seated or lying on your back (leg press), feet should be shoulder wide with toes straight ahead; knees should be bent to a maximum of 90 degrees, and hips flexed to 45–60 degrees.

Motion: Push the weight, keeping your feet flat on the platform, until your knees are nearly straight, then slowly bring the weight back to the starting position.

Back Squat

Muscle groups strengthened: Front of thighs, back of thighs and hips, buttocks, and back

Position: Rest the bar on your upper back with the weight over your hips or midfoot; back should be straight with shoulder blades pulled back toward each other.

Grip: Overhand with thumbs wrapped around bar.

Motion: Straighten both legs to lift the bar off the rack and move away from the rack with the help of spotters. Keeping your back straight and eyes looking forward with feet flat on the floor, bend your knees. Lower the weight until your thighs are parallel to the floor, then rise slowly. (Unless you have a back squat machine, this exercise requires a spotter and expert technique.)

Breathing: Exhale as you lift, inhale, return to the starting position.

3. Latissimus Pull (Figure 12.4)

Muscles strengthened: Upper back, biceps.

Position: Sit or kneel with arms extended, using either a wide or narrow grip (narrow allows for more range of motion).

Grip: Overhand or underhand.

Motion: Slowly pull the bar behind or in front of the lower portion of your neck.

Breathing: Exhale as you pull the bar down, inhale as the bar raises.

4. Leg Curl (Figure 12.5)

Muscles strengthened: Back of the thighs

Position: Seated or lying on your abdomen (depending on the machine); the pads should be at ankle level, pressing against your heel cord (Achilles tendon).

Motion: Flex your knees slowly, until the angle is 90 degrees or greater.

Breathing: Exhale as you flex your knees, inhale as your knees straighten.

TABLE 12.9   **The Muscle-Building Exercises That Work** (*continued*)

5. Shoulder Press (Military Press) (Figure 12.6)
Muscles Strengthened: Shoulders, back of upper arm.
Position: Bar should be about shoulder height, feet flat on the floor, about shoulder width.
Grip: Overhand with thumbs wrapped around the bar.
Motion: Lift the bar up, so it ends directly over the middle of your head.
Breathing: Inhale as you lower the weight, exhale as you raise the bar.

6. Leg Extension (Figure 12.7)
Muscles strengthened: Front of thighs.
Position: Sit in the leg-extension machine with your feet just under the ankle pads.
Motion: Raise the pad until your legs are parallel to the floor, then return to the starting position.
Breathing: Exhale as you raise your legs, inhale as you lower them.

7. Abdominal Crunches (Figure 12.8)
Muscles strengthened: Abdominals.
Position: Lie on your back, knees bent and arms crossed over your chest.
Motion: Slowly curl your chest and head until your shoulder blades are off the floor. Hold for the count of "two" then return to the floor (first day, do 20 crunches, then increase 5 per day). Unlike other strength training, you can do crunches every day.
Breathing: Exhale as you lift up, inhale as you return your shoulder blades to the floor.

8. Arm Curls (Biceps Curls) (Figure 12.9)
Muscles strengthened: Biceps (front of arm)
Position: Elbows extended, hold bar with underhand grip.
Motion: Bring the bar up toward your chest for a count of "two," then slowly lower the bar.
Breathing: Exhale as you flex your elbows, inhale as you extend your arms.

Workout #1

Workout # 1 is a great general SUV conditioning program. You can use this for months. It begins and ends the week with light-to-moderate weights (about 50 percent of the maximum weight you can lift). In mid-week, you increase the weight a small amount and reduce the repetitions for most lifts. The biceps exercise (arm curl) is held constant, because it is the smallest muscle group you exercise and there is little reason to create higher stress on this muscle. As you become stronger and are able to complete all the sets and repetitions, gradually increase the weight.

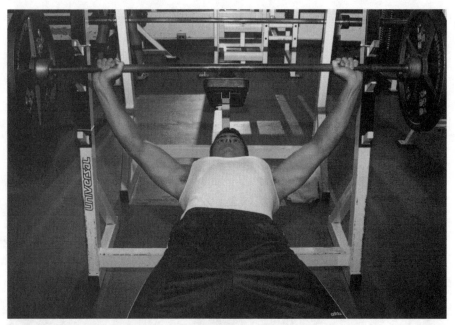

Figure 12.1   The traditional bench press with free weights.

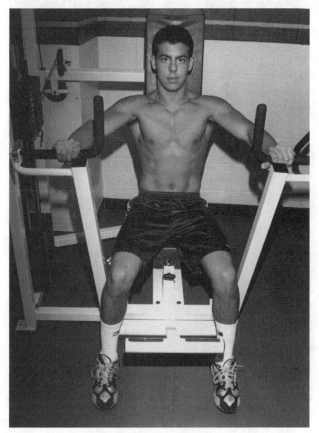

Figure 12.2   A seated machine bench press.

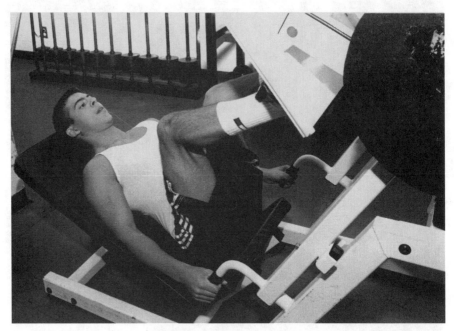

Figure 12.3   Reclining leg press.

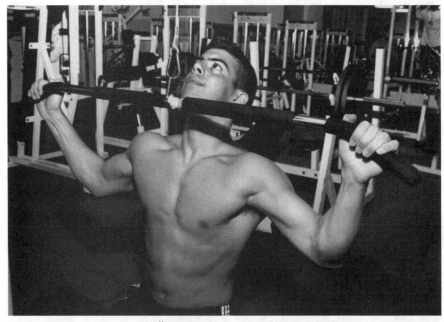

Figure 12.4   Latissimus pull.

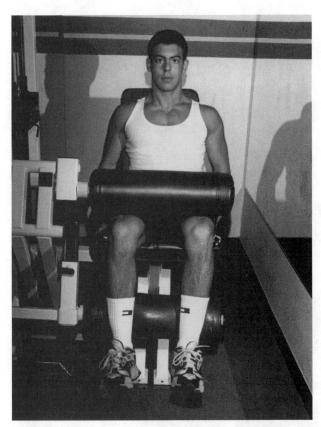

Figure 12.5   Leg curl.

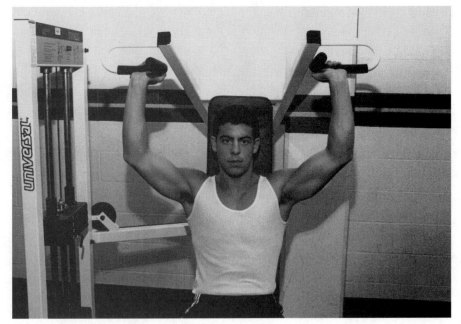

Figure 12.6   Shoulder press.

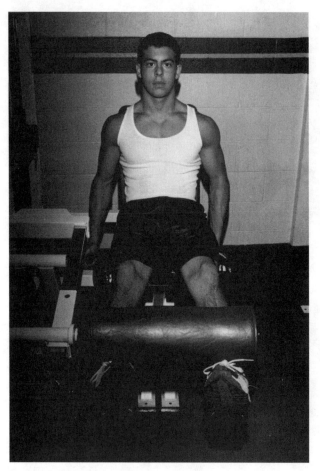

Figure 12.7   Leg extension.

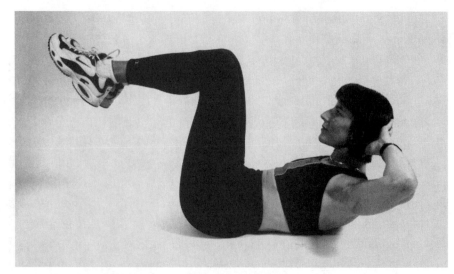

Figure 12.8   Abdominal crunch with hips flexed.

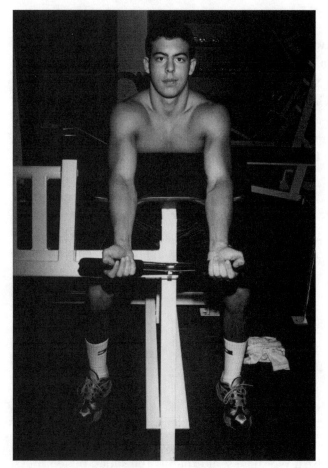

Figure 12.9   The start of the biceps curl.

Exercise	Monday (light-moderate weight)		Wednesday (moderate weight)		Friday (light-moderate weight)	
	Sets	Repetitions	Sets	Repetitions	Sets	Repetitions
Leg press	4	15–20	4	10–12	4	15–20
Bench press	4	12–15	3	8–10	4	12–15
Leg extensions	4	12–15	4	10–12	4	12–15
Shoulder press	3	12–15	3	10–12	3	12–15
Latissimus pull	3	12–15	3	10–12	3	12–15
Leg curl	4	12–15	2	10–12	4	12–15
Arm curl	3	10–12	3	10–12	3	10–12
Crunches	4	20–30	4	20–30	4	20–30

Workout #2

Workout #2 is in between an SUV and a Truck workout. The weights are moderately heavy on each day, but during your midweek workout, you keep the weight the same but reduce the repetitions to give your muscles a little break. This allows your muscles to repair from the heavier workout on Monday and still train at a higher weight. Instead of keeping the weight the same during the Wednesday workout, you could reduce the weight and keep the repetitions the same as on Monday and Friday.

Exercise	Monday (moderate-heavy weight)		Wednesday (moderate-heavy weight)		Friday (moderate-heavy weight)	
	Sets	Repetitions	Sets	Repetitions	Sets	Repetitions
Squat	3	8–12	4	3–4	3	8–12
Bench press	3	6–10	3	3–4	3	6–10
Leg extensions	3	8–12	4	4–6	3	8–12
Shoulder press	3	10–12	3	4–6	3	10–12
Latissimus pull	3	8–12	3	4–6	3	8–12
Leg curl	3	12–15	2	10–12	3	12–15
Arm curl	3	10–12	3	10–12	3	10–12
Crunches	4	20–30	4	20–30	4	20–30

You can split the exercise into a six-day per week training schedule by splitting the exercises. We suggest alternating the squat, bench press, leg extentions, and crunches on Monday, Wednesday, and Friday, with shoulder press, latissimus pull, leg curl, arm curl, and crunches on Tuesday, Thursday, and Saturday. Then take a break on Sunday. As you work one muscle group, the other muscles you trained the day before are repairing and refueling. Your workouts are more frequent, but you can do them in less time. Then add aerobics, either after (our preference) or before your strength training. Photocopy and use the exercise logs in the appendix to record and help guide your training.

Flexibility Exercises

Flexibility exercises have not been closely studied to understand their link with risk factors for heart disease, weight loss, bone strengthening, and lifespan. But, your ability to move your joints freely and without pain through a wide range of motion is important not only to your physical fitness, but for the ability to prevent injury during exercise. Greater flexibility of the spine may go a long way toward preventing back pain. Try the flex test to measure your back and hip flexibility. Repeat this test every few weeks to gauge your improvement.

Flex Testing

(sit and reach)
1. Sit on the floor with a yardstick between your extended legs and with your feet approximately 12 inches apart.
2. Place the yardstick's 15 inch mark at the level of your heels.
3. With your arms outstretched, place your right hand over your left with middle fingers above each other.
4. Bend forward from the waist and slide your fingertips along the yardstick, as far as you can. Repeat three times.
5. Record the highest score, to the nearest inch.

Back Stretch #1 (see Figure 4.5a)

1. Lie on your back
2. Press one or both knees into chest, holding your shinbones with your hands.
3. Release and repeat.

Back Stretch #2 (Figure 12.10)

1. Rest on hands and knees.
2. Dip your back, keeping head up and chin out.
3. Arch your back.

Calf Stretch (Figure 12.11)

1. Stand about a foot from a wall, then extend one leg behind you, keeping both feet flat on the floor, with toes pointed straight ahead, and your rear knee straight.
2. Move your hips forward, keeping lower back flat.
3. Lean into the wall until you feel tension in the calf muscle of the extended leg.
4. Repeat.

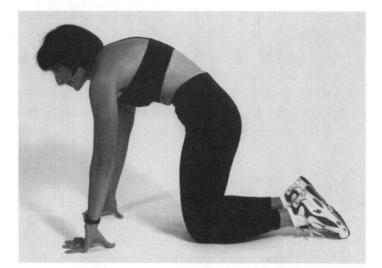

Figure 12.10   Back stretch 2 (back arch phase).

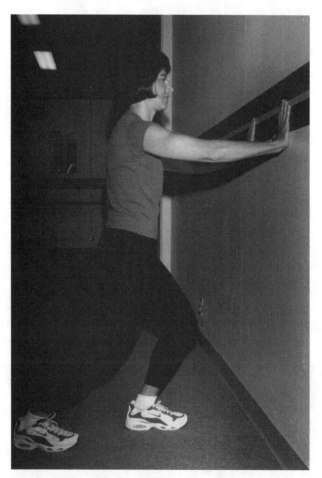

Figure 12.11   Calf stretch.

Achilles Tendon Stretch (Figure 12.12)

1. Get into position for calf stretch.
2. Lower hips downward as you slightly bend the knee of the extended leg.
3. Keep both heels flat on the floor and toes straight ahead.
4. Hold the stretch 10 seconds, then stretch the other leg.
5. Repeat

Note: This area requires only a slight feel of stretching.

General advice: Hold stretches for 10 to 30 seconds without straining or bouncing, which may create or increase muscle tears. Breathe deeply and rhythmically.

Shoulder Stretches

Hold each stretch for 10 to 15 seconds and repeat three times.

Triceps Stretch (Figure 12.13)

1. Cross left arm over chest.
2. Pull left elbow with right hand.
3. Repeat on the other side.

Overhead Triceps Stretch (Figure 12.14)

1. Raise your right arm.
2. Pull left elbow with right hand.
3. Repeat on the other side

   For each of the following stretches, move to the point of slight discomfort, but not so far as to cause pain. Hold each position about 15 to 20 seconds. Stretch slowly while breathing deeply. Repeat each stretch several times on both sides of your body.

Quadriceps Stretch (Figure 12.15)

This stretches the muscle on the front of the thigh that connects to your knee joint.

1. Stand on your left leg.
2. Reach back and hold your right foot behind you with your left hand.
3. Balance against a wall, counter, or chair with your free hand as you pull gently upward on your right foot.

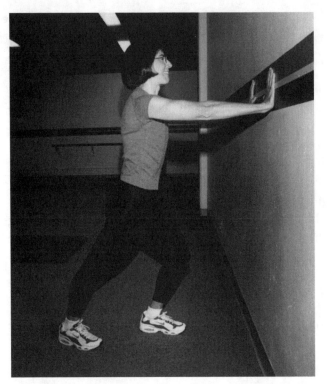

Figure 12.12   Achilles tendon (heel cord) stretch of the right (extended) leg.

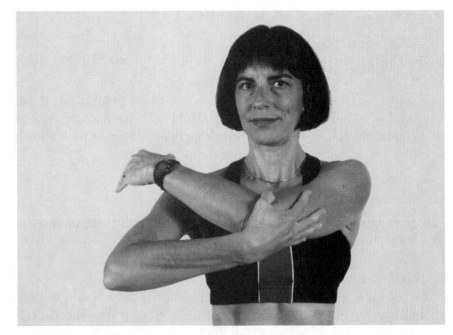

Figure 12.13   Cross-chest triceps stretch.

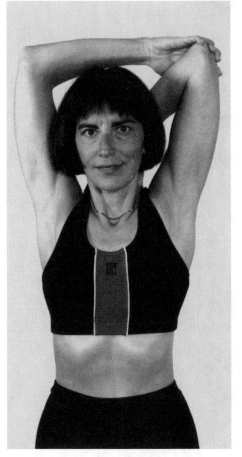

Figure 12.14 Overhead triceps stretch.

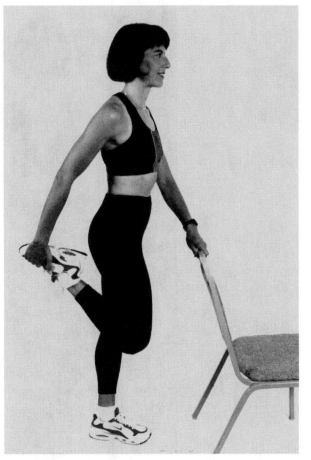

Figure 12.15 Quadriceps (thigh) stretch of the right leg.

4. You should feel a stretch in your right thigh, not in the knee.
5. Reverse and repeat.

Iliotibial Band Stretch (Figure 12.16)

This stretches the iliotibial, or I-T, band, the fibrous tissue on the side of your thigh running from hip to knee.

1. Stand sideways to a wall, leaning against it with your arm or palm of your hand.
2. Move your inside foot behind and to the far side of your stationary foot.

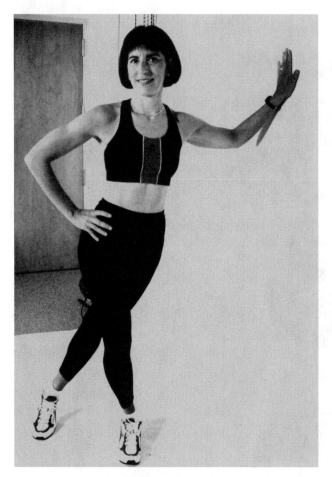

Figure 12.16   Iliotibial band stretch.

3. Lean your hip toward the wall while bending the stationary knee and keeping the other knee straight.
4. Use your free hand to press your body toward the wall.
5. Feel a stretch at the outside of the inside hip and upper thigh.
6. Reverse and repeat.

Final Words

Now you have the tools to gain endurance, strength, and flexibility. Use your talents and begin your journey to better health.

Afterword: Preventing and Treating Common Exercise Problems

Exercise is safe. However, when you challenge your body, injuries can occur to your muscles, tendons, ligaments, and bones. The longer and harder we train and the older our body is, the more likely we are to become injured. Despite what you see on the football field, most injuries during physical activity do not occur all of a sudden. They slowly sneak up on you. At first, you may feel a twinge. Then the discomfort tends to last a little longer and takes longer to heal. We often shrug them off and keep exercising. But if we don't change the way we are exercising, these nagging problems often worsen and become chronic and persistent.

Before getting into specifics, it is important to know two important rules for treatment of wear-and-tear or "overuse injuries." First, when they occur, you will need to cut back on the particular exercise that caused the problem. Trying to work through an injury will make the problem worse. Second, changing your workout will help you keep your fitness and allow the injured body part time to heal. And, third, if the problem does not resolve, get professional help. This way, the health benefits of exercise won't be lost, and you literally won't lose a step.

The people described in this chapter and their problems are not meant to cover every muscle pull, joint ache, or injury contained in a medical textbook. But their stories will give you some insight into some common problems that can arise during your training.

Jack, a 45-year-old banker, is a "weekend warrior." He exercises only when he is in the mood. Participating in softball games on an occasional Saturday and playing basketball at a nearby grade school gym twice each month, Jack never felt like he was getting into shape. The day after he exercised, he was always sore. He dressed slowly in the morning and limped around the office for the next two to three days. In mid-July, his friend Aaron asked Jack to join him for a 15 kilometer fun-run around a local lake. The race started later than usual because of some technical delays, and it was a bright, 72 degrees at race time.

During the first portion of the run, Aaron was surprised how fast Jack was running, despite not training. With his adrenaline pumping, Jack was able to keep up with Aaron for the first two miles. Aaron repeatedly asked him if he wanted to slow the pace, but Jack said that he felt fine and stayed alongside his friend, jogging $7^1/_2$ minutes per mile. To keep up, he did not stop to drink fluid. As the temperature steadily climbed he began to sweat profusely. Jack did not drink much fluid before the race, and the four beers he had the evening before at a friend's barbecue caused him to have a full bladder and a few extra bathroom visits at night.

After about 30 minutes, Jack developed leg cramps and began to feel tired, but he was determined to keep running. He thought the cramping and fatigue would pass. After a few more minutes, Jack began to have some nausea, his head began pounding, but he continued jogging. Finally, Jack told Aaron to run ahead, because he needed to slow down. As Aaron became a smaller and smaller figure in the distance, Jack appeared more like he was running in slow motion. As he staggered across the finish line, his face beet red and no longer sweating, Jack appeared somewhat lost and confused. An alert race volunteer ran over to Jack and assisted him to the emergency medical tent.

Heat Injury and Sweat

Heat is produced as we exercise. The harder we work, the more heat we generate. Also, when the weather or training room is warm, we build up more heat in our body. Your body needs water to cool off, just like an engine needs water in its radiator. If we did not have a cooling system, our body temperature would increase about 1 degree for every 5 minutes of moderate exercise.

How do we keep our body cool during exercise? Perspiration and evaporation of our sweat are the major ways we avoid excess body temperature, with some extra heat lost through rapid breathing. In fact, those who train in the heat develop more efficient cooling systems as they become acclimated to the environment; they can sweat nearly twice as much as those not accustomed to warmer temperatures.

Hot and humid weather makes it more difficult for us to lose the build-up of body heat when we exercise. The warmer temperatures cause more water loss, while the humidity reduces evaporation of water from our skin because the air is already saturated with water.

You can add insult to this process, as Jack did, by drinking alcohol. Although you might think that beer would quench your thirst, alcohol causes more fluid to be lost in the urine, because of its ability to reduce the pituitary gland's output of a hormone called antidiuretic hormone. This causes extra urine flow and loss of water and accounts for the next morning's thirst and dry mouth.

Jack was a set-up for heat injury. First, he was not conditioned for running. Because of his lack of training, his body was not an efficient cooling machine. Fitter people actually sweat more, which makes it easier to get rid of excess heat production during exercise. Jack's use of alcohol the night before his race left him somewhat depleted of body water, even before the race began. Because he didn't drink much fluid prior to or during the run, his dehydration quickly worsened. This reduced his ability to sweat and cool off.

Regular training, avoiding exercise during the hottest time of the day, drinking enough fluid, and recognizing the early symptoms of heat illness are the best way to avoid heat related injury. Table A.1 lists the major types of heat illness, the symptoms, and skin appearance.

Treatment of heat illness includes getting the person to a cool, shaded area and correcting his or her dehydration by giving him or her fluids. Soaking the body with water and using a fan can speed up the

Dogs do not sweat. They get rid of heat by rapid, short pants. In the summer, humans stay cool by sweating and wearing short pants.

Conditions that make you more prone to heat injury include low fitness level, not being acclimated to heat, pregnancy, use of diuretics (water pills), and certain antidepressant medications.

Measuring temperature by using an oral thermometer may underestimate core body temperature, which is better assessed by use of a rectal thermometer. Core body temperature is at least one or more degrees higher.

TABLE A.1 **Heat Injury**

Condition	Body Temperature	Symptoms	Skin Appearance
Heat cramps	About 101 degrees F	Muscle cramps	Sweaty
Heat exhaustion	About 102 degrees F	Chills, weakness, headache, dizziness, and nausea	Flushed and very sweaty
Heat stroke	Above 104 degrees F	Confusion, feeling lightheaded, loss of consciousness, convulsions (seizures)	Red, hot, and dry (no sweat)

cooling process. In the more severe cases, packing part or all of the body in ice can be effective.

Do the following to avoid heat injuries:

- Drink about 16 ounces (2 cups) of water before exercise, even if you are not thirsty.
- Your urine should be light yellow or colorless before exercise.
- Drink about 1 cup of water every 20 minutes when you exercise. In warmer weather (over 80 degrees), drink more.
- Take frequent breaks from exercise in hot weather.
- Train in the morning or late afternoon when the temperature is cooler (before 10:00 A.M. or after 5:00 P.M.).
- Be a cool dresser. Wear only lightweight clothes made of porous materials that breathe.

In the tent, Jack's oral temperature was measured at 103 degrees. The physicians decided Jack was suffering from heat injury and began treating him by pouring cool water all over his body and providing him with cool liquids to drink. Ice was packed under his armpits and around his groin. The air from a large portable fan was directed at Jack. Over the next 30 minutes, his temperature slowly returned to normal.

Thirst and Exercise

Our thirst doesn't always tell us how dehydrated we are, especially when we exercise. So, never rely on how thirsty you feel when deciding when and how much to drink. The harder you work, the more water you lose. Drink before, during, and after you train. At extreme temperatures with high humidity, you may need to drink more than one-half-gallon of fluid every hour and take breaks every 10 minutes to stave off the ravages of heat. Perform this simple check to see how you are doing. Weigh yourself before and after your workout. For each pound lost, you needed to drink 2 full cups (16 ounces) of fluid.

What to Drink

You may be wondering which type of drink is best. Do you need a highly advertised sports drink? Will a sports drink help your performance? The answer is that when you exercise less than one hour, even if the training is vigorous, all you need is water.

If you feel hot, you are too hot.

If you can't stand the heat, stay out of the kitchen.—Harry S. Truman

Sports drinks are mainly water with a little bit of sugar and salt added. Most are tasty and may stimulate you to drink more fluid. This can help you avoid dehydration and heat illness. Also, if you are exercising more than one hour, the sugar in a sports drink can give you extra carbohydrate to aid your performance. Otherwise, we recommend drinking good old H_2O.

Do not drink soft drinks or fruit juices during exercise. Soft drinks have 11 percent carbohydrate and typically have carbonation, while fruit juices often contain 12 percent or more in sugars. Carbonation can result in bloating and nausea, and high concentrations of sugar will reduce the speed of fluid absorption. Sports beverages generally contain about 8 percent or less carbohydrate, which actually helps you absorb water.

If you want to make an inexpensive sports drink, dilute apple juice or other fruit juices with an equal amount of water. This will lower the concentration of the sugar in the drink and replenish your fluid losses during exercise.

> Sports drinks can be helpful if you are exercising vigorously for more than an hour. But water usually is all you need to drink before, during, and after exercise. And it's free from the tap.

> Never use salt tablets. This can worsen the effect of dehydration,

Injuries

Foot Problems

Sonia, a 58-year-old pharmacist, exercised by walking on her treadmill for 45 minutes each day. She started exercising to keep trim, but found that with her workouts she could eliminate one of the three medicines needed to treat her hard-to-control blood pressure. Over the past six weeks, she began to have pain in her left heel. Now the right heel was hurting, too, and just walking was becoming difficult. She tried new walking shoes, but this did not reduce the pain. After another week of limping through her daily treadmill walks, she decided to see a physician.

The most common foot problem among exercisers is plantar fasciitis (fash-ee-eye-tis). The plantar fascia is a wide band of fibrous tissue that connects the heel to the base of the toes on the undersurface of the foot. Nearly 80 percent of heel pain is due to inflammation of this fascia. It can be a very painful condition, often caused by overuse and, unfortunately, by getting older. Also, excessive exercise, rapid weight gain, and either a very high arch or flat feet can lead to plantar fasciitis. Many times a heel spur, which is a small protrusion of bone from your heel due to repeated trauma, is associated with the pain and inflammation. With this condition, walking on your toes or just pushing off with your toes as you walk will stretch the fascia and make the pain worse. Sometimes the inflamed tissue can squeeze a small nerve (the lateral plantar nerve), resulting in numbness on the outer portion of the sole of your foot.

If you keep trying to work through the pain of plantar fasciitis, your pain and disability can be prolonged and last up to a year or more.

Treatment of Plantar Fasciitis

Recognition and early treatment are important. For more immediate treatment of the pain and inflammation, ice your heel for 10 minutes, five or more times each day, and wear a heel cup to cushion the inflamed area. Begin wearing shoes with rigid soles to prevent the bottom of your foot from overstretching. Also, gentle stretching and over-the-counter orthotic devices (foot supports) are helpful in treating plantar fasciitis. In fact, one study showed that slowly stretching your foot several minutes a day is as effective as the custom fit, expensive foot supports (orthotics). Strengthening the muscles of your arch by curling your toes can help. (Here is a simple exercise: Place a towel on a floor that is not carpeted. Sit on a chair, placing your feet on the towel. Curl your toes as if you were pulling the towel towards you. Do this for 3 to 5 minutes, three times each day.) While recovering, participate only in exercises that do not stress the sole of your foot. Cycling and rowing can be great alternative ways to train. Because you will be sitting, you are removing most of the weight stress from your feet, eliminating tension on the plantar fascia.

Only 2 percent of heel spurs and plantar fasciitis will require surgery.

In more severe cases, a cortisone injection into the fascia at the heel can be helpful. Physical therapy, using ultrasound, which results in high-frequency sound vibrations, creates deep heat therapy, while muscular stimulation using a physical therapy device called a galvanic stimulator may speed recovery. Rarely, surgery is necessary, but this is more likely to occur if a heel spur is present.

Ankle Sprains

Who hasn't had an ankle sprain? If you have participated in sports or regular exercise, you can probably insert your story of an ankle sprain in this book. The ankle is one of the most frequently injured joints for those who participate in sports. In fact, injuries to the ankle represent about one out of every five injuries!

Your ankle (Figure A.1) includes the bottom of the shin bone (the tibia), representing the inner portion of the ankle, the smaller leg bone (the fibula), the outer portion of the ankle, and the Talus bone of the foot. There are three major ligaments of the ankle that hold these bones together. These ligaments also allow ankle motion, but only within certain limits.

An ankle sprain is an injury of one of the supporting ligaments, usually due to overstretching or tearing. This more often occurs in sports where there is side-to-side movement, such as basketball, soccer, tennis, squash, and racquetball. But it occurs in other activities, especially when the ground is uneven and the ankle turns on itself. When this occurs, there is pain, blood vessels can rupture and bleed around the joint, and the ankle becomes less stable. Also, tendons from the muscles of the leg can be stretched and damaged, and a fracture of the ends of the tibia and/or fibula and the metatarsal foot bones can occur.

There are three different levels of ankle sprains, based on the severity of damage. Returning to the activity should be done only when

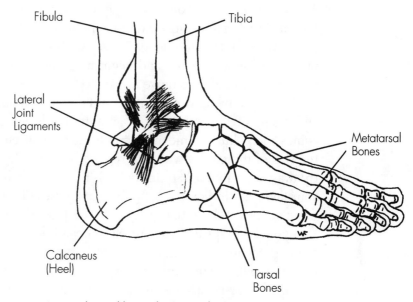

Figure A.1   The ankle and surrounding structures.

you are pain free, have regained a full range of motion, and have sufficient ankle strength. It is very important to strengthen your ankle after a sprain to help prevent another ankle injury.

Grade I ankle sprains involve excessive stretching of one or more ankle ligaments, but the ligament is not torn. Usually blood vessels are not damaged, and there is no bruising around your ankle. Rest, icing the ankle with a compression bandage (like an ace wrap), and elevating your ankle on several pillows is all that is necessary. When the sprain first occurs, apply the ice for 10 to 15 minutes, then allow another 10 to 15 minutes to pass without ice. Reapply the ice to your ankle, off and on for 10 to 15 minutes for the next several hours. This is called RICE therapy (rest, ice, compression, elevation), and it will reduce swelling and limit pain. The time of recovery depends on the extent of the damage. Usually a few days to two weeks of healing are needed, followed by ankle strengthening and stretching exercises.

A *grade II* ankle sprain means there is a tear of one or more of your ankle ligaments, but the ankle is not unstable. Some ligaments of your leg are often injured or torn. Bleeding occurs with this injury and you will see bluish bruising by one day after the sprain. RICE therapy should be the initial treatment, similar to grade I sprains. However, for many grade II sprains, a removable splint or brace that prevents excessive side-to-side ankle movement is often used for four to five days. Avoid placing weight on your injured ankle if there is significant pain. Use of crutches for a few days may help speed the healing process by giving your ankle some needed rest. As the ankle pain diminishes, remove the splint or brace and begin range of motion exercises. But do not force your ankle to move in pain.

Start by moving your joint up and down, as if you were stepping on and easing off the gas pedal of an automobile. As your ankle joint becomes more limber, moving your foot in small circles and increasing the size of the circles will help restore mobility. As healing progresses, try drawing numbers (1 through 9) in the air with your toes, keeping your knee and hip motionless. Other exercises (Table A.2) can be done, using surgical tubing that is available at most drug and athletic stores. A physical therapist or your physician can help you initiate this type of training. Swimming is a great way to improve strength and aid in ankle flexibility before you attempt running or participation in other sports.

Grade III sprains are the most severe: you have ligament tear and an unstable ankle. A physician needs to immobilize your ankle joint.

TABLE A.2 **Exercises to Strengthen Your Ankles**

1. While sitting in a chair, loop one end of the elastic tubing around the ball of your foot, keeping your heel on the floor and hold the ends of the tubing in your hand. Push on the tubing with the ball of your foot as if you are stepping on the gas pedal of your automobile. Repeat this 10 times, rest for 60 seconds. Do this four times, three times each day. Increase the number of repetitions as your ankle strength improves.

2. Tie the surgical tubing in a knot and place it around the leg of a table. Sit on a chair and loop the surgical tubing around the top of your foot, just below your toes, keeping your heel on the floor. Pull back your foot, as if you were easing off the gas pedal of your automobile, keeping tension on the tubing. Repeat this 10 times, rest for 60 seconds. Do this four times, three times each day. Increase the number of repetitions as your ankle strength improves.

3. Take the tied surgical tubing, as in exercise 2 and loop it around the leg of a table. Sit on a chair, looping the tubing around the outside of your foot just below your toes, keeping your foot flat on the floor. Stretch the tubing by moving your foot sideways, away from your other leg using your heel as a pivot. Then place the loop around the inside of your foot, just below your toes, keeping your foot flat on the floor. Stretch the tubing by moving your foot sideways toward your other leg, using your heel as a pivot. As in exercises 1 and 2, perform each exercise 10 times and repeat three more times, four times each day, increasing the number of repetitions as your ankle strength improves.

The ankle is usually positioned so as to enhance correct healing of the ligaments. A walking cast is often used, with weight placed on the cast as tolerated. After the cast is removed, about three weeks later, rehabilitation of the ankle is started to regain motion and strength. In addition, because we can lose the sense of where our ankle is after a severe ankle sprain, specialized exercises are used with a shifting flat surface, known as a BAPS, or biomechanic ankle proprioceptive system board, as one of the rehabilitation devices. This type of exercise can help you prevent your next ankle sprain. Swimming before weight-bearing exercise often is recommended. This will aid ankle flexibility and strengthening, without excessive stress.

Remember, you should be pain free with normal ankle movement before progressing to other conditioning exercises such as rope skipping and jogging on level ground. Surgery is rarely needed after ankle sprains, but may be necessary to repair severely damaged ligaments and tendons.

To prevent recurrent ankle injuries in the future, ankle supports, or wearing high-top athletic shoes can help. This is especially true for activities that call for rapid changes in direction or training on uneven ground. If you have had ankle sprains before, prevent recurrent problems by using an ankle support along with ankle-strengthening exercises.

Knee and Lower Leg Injuries

Keith is a 45-year-old physician who quit playing basketball three years ago. He stopped participating because there were too many games in which friends would grab their knee or ankle and be carried off to the emergency room. Some required surgery. As Keith put it, "the risk-to-benefit ratio was getting too high. Only if I were making a million dollars a year would the benefit be much greater than the risk. Even scoring 30 points each game would not mean as much to me as the risk of surgery."

Two days ago, while at a medical convention in Texas, Keith was exercising in the hotel gym. A medical student attending the conference challenged him to join in a basketball game in an adjoining court. Against his better judgement, Keith agreed to participate. He felt great playing again. His first two shots went in without touching the backboard . . . swish. The third outside shot bounced high off the rim, and he rushed toward the basket to get the rebound. Jumping in the air and grabbing the ball with both hands, he came down to earth with a thud, landing on a teammate's foot. He felt a snap in his right knee that made him wince. But he had to finish the game, and in the process, he scored the winning bucket.

Afterward, he limped to the dressing room and showered. His knee felt stiff and was becoming more painful. Looking down, he noticed it was swollen to more than twice its previous size. He thought about his former risk-benefit rule and shook his head.

Your knees are unique structures. The knee actually consists of three joints. Two separate joints are between the two smooth ends of your femur or thigh bone. Each connects with the two surfaces of your tibia, the larger of the two bones of the lower leg. The third joint is between your femur and kneecap, known as the patella.

Your knees take the impact of your weight as you walk, run, or jump. Although the knee is stabilized by ligaments that connect the bones of the knee joint, without the powerful muscles of your legs, especially the large quadriceps of the thigh, your knee would be very unstable and unable to support most athletic activities (Figure A.2).

Special stray fiber band ligaments help hold the knee together. Two major ligaments (the medial and lateral collateral ligaments) support

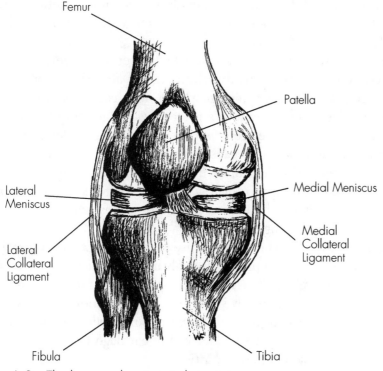

Femur

Patella

Lateral Meniscus

Medial Meniscus

Lateral Collateral Ligament

Medial Collateral Ligament

Fibula

Tibia

Figure A.2 The knee and associated structures.

the surrounding portions of the knee, while two internal knee liga-ments (the anterior cruciate and posterior cruciate) prevent the thigh bone from slipping forward or backward on the shin bone. Two smooth shock absorbing cartilage pads known as menisci sit between your tibia and the slick cartilage-covered condyles of the femur. The menisci and condyles form a smooth surface, reducing friction between your thigh and leg bone, enabling you to bend and straighten your knee joint without stiffness.

Knee Cartilage (Meniscus) Injury

As we age, our cartilage becomes more brittle. With repeated stress, joint cartilage can be damaged by wear and tear, and small breaks or tears can develop. However, with sudden impact, it can be ripped. Keith tore his right (medial) inside meniscus. He made his own diagno-sis, based on the fact that he could barely bend his knee and had pain when he pressed the small space between his femur and tibia with his thumb. Specialized scanning, known as magnetic resonance imaging (MRI), confirmed the diagnosis.

An acutely torn meniscus is usually treated by surgery. Today this procedure can be performed with the aid of an arthroscope (a hand-held, long, surgical joint microscope) in most cases. Occasionally, the surgeon needs only to remove a piece of cartilage, but sometimes removal of the entire meniscus is necessary. Young athletes may have their meniscus repaired because there is a better chance of healing. But, as we become older our cartilage is less likely to repair itself after the tear is stitched. Approximately seven days after surgery, rehabilitation is started, first with range-of-motion exercises, and followed by cycling and strengthening.

For meniscus tears due to overuse and degeneration, surgery is not always necessary. If you participate only in low-impact activities such as swimming or cycling, it is safe to continue your exercise. For many people, the symptoms resolve with time. If discomfort remains, a specific knee brace can be helpful. However some will eventually require surgery to smooth out the surface of the cartilage to reduce pain and prevent the development of arthritis.

The meniscus of your knee has no blood supply. So, if it becomes damaged, it does not heal as well as other tissues. As we age, the meniscus naturally degenerates and can more easily tear with stress. Torn pieces can prevent the normal movement of the knee, causing pain, swelling, and reducing motion, occasionally causing it to "lock" in one position.

Keith had arthroscopic surgery as an outpatient when he returned home. His surgeon removed a portion of the meniscus. He used crutches for two days, then began walking without assistance. Within a week , Keith and his wife went to Vancouver, British Columbia, for their anniversary. He walked all over the city and rode a bike through the park for daily rehabilitation. He began jogging two months later. Eight years after surgery, he continues to exercise regularly but has avoided any competitive basketball games, although he will challenge his 11-year-old son, Alex, to a game of HORSE.

Knee Ligament Injury

Other structures in Keith's knee could have been damaged during the game. Once, the most-feared injury by athletes was a tear of the knee's anterior cruciate ligament (ACL). This short fibrous band connects the thigh bone or femur and your shin bone (tibia). By its attachment, it prevents your leg from sliding too far forward, in front of your thigh. About half of the time, an ACL tear is accompanied with a torn meniscus. Sort of an unfortunate two-for-one deal. In the past, ACL injuries ended the athletic careers of many athletes. However, newer surgical reconstruction and rehabilitation methods have allowed athletes to return to their sport and perform at the highest levels.

When an ACL injury occurs, the person can often hear a pop as the ligament tears. This is followed by considerable pain. Unlike Keith, who continued playing basketball, those with an anterior cruciate ligament tear cannot continue to play. They usually have to be carried off the court, because the knee becomes so unstable it cannot bear any weight. Despite how it sounds, not all ACL tears need surgery. This is true especially if you are not going to perform activities that require quick turns and pivoting motion. People can jog, ride a bike, and use a rowing machine without an ACL. If you want to participate in recreational sports that are not too competitive, a knee brace can be used successfully.

However, for activities that require turning and twisting with cleats, and if you plan to participate in competitive athletics, surgical repair of the ACL is recommended. Reconstructive surgery most often involves use of a person's own tendon, often taken from the back of the thigh. Occasionally a tendon from another person is used and inserted between the knee joint to replace the torn ligament. After physical therapy, competitive athletics can resume.

Pain at the Third Joint of the Knee

The undersurface of your kneecap, or patella, is part of the knee joint. When the kneecap does not track or move correctly, a portion of this surface comes under excessive stress and may soften. This condition is known as chondromalacia, or runner's knee, and it results in pain. The discomfort is often felt at the inner side of the knee or just below the kneecap. Pain can worsen after sitting for a long time with your knees bent, by jogging downhill, or while walking down stairs. Because of their anatomy or how they run, some people are more prone to develop chondromalacia. This includes women with wide hips, those with a weak muscle of the inner thigh (the vastus medialis), runners who pronate their feet (turning their foot toward the inside of their sole) as they jog, and people with a malpositioned kneecap.

When the cause of chondromalacia is due to a malpositioned or poorly tracking patella, straight leg raises with or without weights (Figure A.3) to strengthen the vastus medialis muscle are prescribed. After

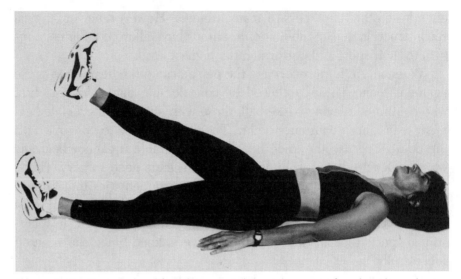

Figure A.3   Straight leg lift without weights as treatment for chondromalacia.

these exercises, icing the knee for 10 to 20 minutes can reduce pain and swelling. A specialized brace can be worn to help the patella move correctly. Stretching the back of your thigh (the hamstrings), low back, and calf (Figures 12.10 and 12.11) can help reduce stress on the knee.

Another Pain In The Leg

Kathy, a 42-year-old mother of three, began jogging 12 weeks ago. She quickly increased her running distances and speed until the past 10 days. After a particularly easy four mile run, she began to feel pain in both legs a few inches below the knee. It became difficult for her to walk for several hours after the jog. Limping around the house for nearly a day, the pain slowly subsided, allowing her to run again. However, following each jog the pains in her legs seemed to last a little longer, and it took more time for Kathy to feel better. She decided to visit her physician when she could not run more than a mile without the pain limiting her exercise.

There are many causes of leg (below the knee and above the ankle) pain. A common pain that occurs with running, especially among those who are new joggers, is shin splints. But new joggers are not the only people who develop this problem. Runners who substantially increase their mileage or change running surfaces can experience this pain, too. Although there is some debate about what really constitutes shin splints, most believe the cause is small tearing of the anterior tibial muscle, away from the bone. Your anterior tibial muscle extends from the midportion of the foot and travels up the front of the leg, inserting just below the knee. It is located at the inside portion of your leg, in front of the calf.

Beginning runners who progress too quickly by running too many miles or too fast, just like Kathy, develop shin splints because they have not allowed their muscles time to build and adapt to the new exercise. Some people, because of the way they run, improperly turn their foot as they hit the ground. Running on the inside (excessive pronation) or the outside (excessive supination) of the foot, can also lead to shin splints. This type of running is a biomechanical problem that is diagnosed by observing the way you run. However, you might be able to diagnose this running problem by just looking at the soles of your jogging shoes. Normal wear of the shoe is to have the outside portion of the heel wear a little more. If the wear is excessive, you run with excessive supination. If the wear is greater on the inside of the heal, then there is too much pronation.

Symptoms of shin splints include a dull aching sensation at the inner portion of the lower leg that occurs during or after jogging. Once the symptoms begin, nearly any leg activity can aggravate the pain. To treat shin splints you need to remove the underlying problem that caused the shin splints in the first place, but to reduce pain and start the healing process, follow the treatment in Table A.3.

This therapy is referred to as RICE. By resting (R), you allow the muscle tears to heal. Icing (I), usually by a compression (C) bandage, reduces the inflammation and pain, and elevation (E) of your leg decreases swelling. Anti-inflammatory medications such as aspirin, ibuprofen, or naproxen also can help relieve pain and swelling.

The long-term treatment of shin splints is designed to reduce your risk of developing the problem again. If you don't have a biomechanical problem and just ran too hard, too fast, you can start by strengthening

---

TABLE A.3   **Immediate Treatment of Shin Splints**

- Rest! Stop jogging
- Ice your legs with a compression (Ace) wrap
- Elevate your legs
- Take anti-inflammatory medication if necessary

your anterior tibial muscles. Elevate your big toe and front portion of the foot upward toward your knee, as if you were easing your foot off the gas pedal of your car. If you do not have any pain while performing this maneuver, add some resistance by placing a towel or surgical tubing over your foot and having a partner hold the ends of the towel or tubing as you raise your foot (Figure A.4). Initially, the resistance should be very light. Perform this exercise 10 to 20 times, three times each day, increasing the number of repetitions every three to four days. After the resistance exercise, stretch the muscles by pulling back on your forefoot and count to 10. Follow this by pushing the forefoot down and count to 10. Repeat this 10 times.

When you restart your jogging, make sure you increase your mileage slowly. Kathy's mistake was the fact that she was progressing

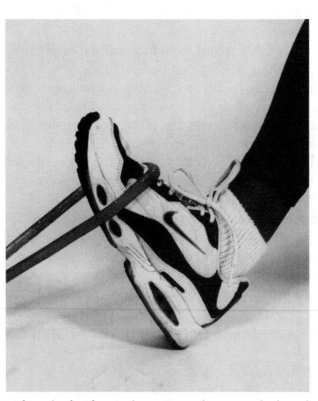

Figure A.4   Lifting the forefoot with resistance by surgical tubing looped over the front of the shoe strengthens lower leg (anterior tibial) muscles.

too fast, beyond the ability of her muscles to adapt. If you have a problem with excessive pronation or supination, you should have orthotics prescribed to control the movement of your ankle as you walk or run. Most successful rehabilitation takes about three months.

Beyond Shin Splints

Two other problems (see Table A.4) can have similar symptoms and at times can be difficult to distinguish from shin splints. This includes stress fractures (also discussed on pages 46–47, Chapter 3). The pain can be similar. A stress fracture is a very small crack in a normal bone. It is not like the typical fracture that occurs with high-impact trauma from an accident. This type of fracture usually occurs after repeated small amounts of trauma or stress on a bone. If the period of rest is insufficient, the bone becomes so weakened that a small break occurs. If the stress is continued, and you continue to exercise in spite of the pain, this can lead to a full break in the bone.

Often the break is so small that an X ray cannot detect any abnormality. But, pressure over the bone where the small break occurred causes pain. This is different from the pain of shin splints, where the discomfort covers a broader area, rather than tenderness at one small point. The diagnosis is usually confirmed by magnetic resonance

TABLE A.4 **Lower Leg Pain**

Problem	Location of Pain	Quality of Pain	Special Features
Shin splints	Along the inside border of the tibia bone, about two-thirds of the way down the lower leg.	Dull ache that occurs during a run.	Pain persists beyond the time of exercise, often 24 or more hours.
Stress fracture	On the bone (tibia) itself; usually you can point to the pain	Sharp pain that gradually increases with more activity.	Can have point tenderness at the site of the fracture.
Compartment syndrome	The outer portion of the lower leg	Dull and deep pain	Initially, the pain resolves after exercise. There can be loss of function, with nerve damage and foot drop.

imaging or a bone scan. The treatment for stress fracture is RICE, but occasionally a cast and crutches are necessary to allow healing.

Another cause of lower leg pain that needs close attention is referred to as compartment syndrome. Although some physicians may refer to this type of pain as shin splints, it can become a more serious problem. Whereas the pain of shin splints usually occurs on the inside portion of your leg, the discomfort of compartment syndrome is most often on the outside area of the shin. Also, unlike Kathy's shin splints, with pain persisting for a day or longer, the pain of compartment syndrome diminishes soon after the exercise stops, unless it is severe.

There are four compartments of the lower leg. These compartments are like stiff tubular socks that extend up the leg. Muscles, nerves, and blood vessels are contained in each compartment. Compartment syndrome occurs when the muscle expands during exercise, due to engorgement of blood and becomes too large for the compartment. The main muscle involved in compartment syndrome of the lower leg due to running is the tibialis posterior muscle, but other muscles can be involved, when other compartments are involved. As the muscle expands, blood vessels are choked and nerves become squished. Pain is due to decreased blood flow and swelling, while nerve compression can cause pain and numbness.

RICE therapy can be helpful immediately. However, at times the swelling is so severe or the compartment is so small that the nerves traveling through the anterior compartment lose their function and lead to a floppy foot; the person begins to lose the ability to bring his or her toes and front of the foot up toward the direction of the knee. In very severe cases, the muscle tissue can be starved for blood because of the pressure build-up, causing gangrene. When this occurs, emergency surgery is necessary to reduce muscle and nerve injury.

Surgery often is performed for competitive athletes with recurrent compartment syndrome. With this surgery, most often the portion of the leg known as the anterior compartment is surgically decompressed, so the muscles have more room to expand.

Hip Problems

Jeff could not sleep because of the pain near his hip. He had started a run-walk exercise program three months ago, but had to stop all exercise be-

If leg pain or numbness persists beyond 24 hours without diminishing, seek medical advice.

cause he experienced pain just after jogging and walking, and now the discomfort was increasing. The pain was on the outside of his upper thigh and would occasionally travel down the outside of his thigh, ending just above the knee. It was hard to get in a comfortable position. Movement in and out of his car and just changing positions from sitting to standing were becoming so painful that he would rather stand in meetings than sit. Jeff finally went to his physician, not because of the hip pain, but because of stomach discomfort after using ibuprofen three to four times each day for the past month. His physician located the pain at the upper portion of his thigh, where the hip joint moves. Pressing with his thumb, Jeff felt that the pain was similar, but movement of his hip joint was normal.

Many people do not recognize that hip joint problems do not occur in the buttocks or the outer thigh. Hip joint pain typically is felt as a pain in the groin or the upper inner thigh, near the crease. Pinpoint pain at the upper outer thigh, near the area at which your thigh pivots, is the area of the joint's bursa. When the bursa becomes inflamed by an acute injury or by overuse, the condition is known as bursitis.

A bursa is a fluid-filled structure that reduces friction between different body tissues. Bursae, in general, are located next to tendons of large joints, such as the hips, shoulders, knees, and elbows.

There are two major hip bursae that can become inflamed, with stiffness and pain developing around the hip joint. Located on the side of the upper thigh, your trochanteric bursa is separated from the actual hip joint by tissue and bone. Trochanteric bursitis caused Jeff's tenderness of the outer hip area. This pain is often sharp or burning and can be made worse with lying on the involved side, climbing stairs, or in some cases, just walking.

The second major bursa of the hip is the ischial bursa. When inflamed, this bursa, located in the upper buttock, causes a dull pain that becomes even more noticeable when you walk uphill or when you sit on hard surfaces for a long time. Treatment includes ice compresses, rest, and anti-inflammatory medications such as aspirin and ibuprofen and sometimes other pain relief medications. Occasionally, bursitis requires needle aspiration of the bursa fluid so it can be sent to the laboratory for further analysis, to make sure there is no infection.

Trochanteric bursitis is commonly seen among middle-aged and older people. Treatment includes rest, ice, and low back and hip stretching. A cortisone injection, physical therapy, and ultrasound treatment by a physiotherapist can be helpful. Surgery is a last resort.

Jeff was treated with an injection of cortisone-like medication into the swollen bursa, with relief of pain. Eight years later, he is doing well and jogging regularly.

Tennis Elbow

Jerry loved tennis. He played every Tuesday, Thursday, and Saturday morning. When he could fit it into his busy real estate agency director's schedule, Jerry played just about any other day, too. At 44 years of age, he had not lost a step. His serve was strong, his backhand accurate, and he was still quick and agile. Although Jerry had won many tournaments, he had the most pleasure just playing with friends. Over the past few weeks, he began to feel a slight twinge at the outside portion of his upper arm, near the elbow. It wasn't enough to stop him from playing, but he felt it, especially when gripping his racquet tightly and using his backhand. The discomfort increased after spending a Sunday afternoon helping his neighbor build a deck. He had to stop hammering with his right hand, and use his left arm to tap in the nails. The following day, while coaching his son's basketball team, Jerry asked the assistant coach, who was a physician, about his problem.

"First, stop playing tennis!" replied the physician-coach. "If you want to play tennis in six to eight weeks, take some time off and ice your elbow."

Did Jerry take the doctor's advice and stop playing tennis?

Jerry had tendinitis of the lateral epicondyle, better known as tennis elbow. This condition is caused by continual small strains and microscopic tears of tissue near the elbow, resulting in inflammation and pain. (And yes, ten*din*itis is correctly spelled ten*din*, not ten*don*, when you add *itis*.) Specifically, the tendon and muscles (especially the extensor carpi radialis muscle) that extend the wrist by bending your hand back, as if you were to push against the wall, are affected. It commonly occurs while playing tennis because of overextension of the wrist during a backhand stroke. But you do not have to play tennis to develop tennis elbow. You can cause lateral epicondylitis by wielding a hammer or other tool. It is the repeated motion over time that eventually causes the injury. This is why people who are in their forties and fifties are more likely to develop tennis elbow.

Tennis Elbow Therapy

Treatment starts with rest, ice, and gentle stretching (Table A.5). Using a forearm (tennis elbow) band that slips around the upper forearm (Figure A.5) takes tension off of the elbow and can reduce discomfort. Pain can last from a few days to a few weeks. Occasionally, anti-inflammatory

TABLE A.5 **Nonsurgical Treatment of Tennis Elbow**

- Rest! Avoid any activity that will overuse the elbow.
- Ice the area just below and to the side of the elbow.
- Compress your forearm with a support band, just below the elbow.
- Gently stretch the wrist.
- Take anti-inflammatory medication and pain relieving drugs.
- Physiotherapy treatment, including heat and/or ultrasound therapy can aid rehabilitation.
- Occasionally an injection of a cortisone (steroid) can help (but never more than three injections).
- Strengthen the muscles and tendons that move wrist using light weights.

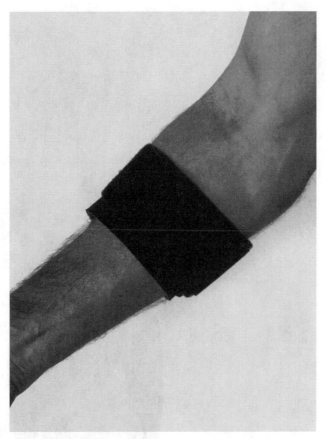

Figure A.5   Tennis elbow forearm sleeve.

medications such as ibuprofen and naproxen can be used. A cortisone injection can be helpful in some cases, but should be reserved for the persistent pain that last more than six weeks, and it must not be done more than three times. There always is a risk of tendon rupture and breakdown of surrounding tissues as a result of a cortisone injection. After the inflammation subsides, heat, massage, and ultrasound treatment by a physiotherapist can speed up the rehabilitation process.

After the pain is relieved, it is important to prevent future recurrences of tennis elbow. This is first done by gently stretching the muscles and tendons of the forearm. Slowly pull back the fingers and wrist into an extended position (like you would push against a wall), then pull the fingers down and back into a fully flexed position. Each stretch should last about 10 seconds and is repeated between 8 and 12 times, three to

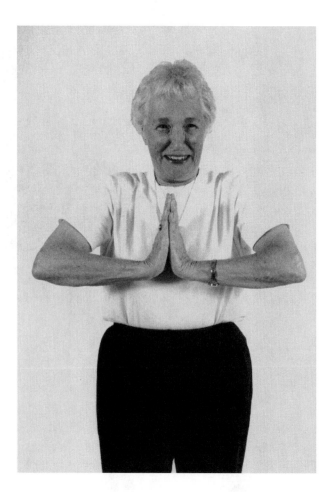

Figure A.6　Wrist extension (praying) stretch for tennis elbow.

four times every day. This stretch should not be painful. So if it hurts, don't do it! Another way to perform these two stretches is to place your hands together, as if you are praying (Figure A.6) and elevate your elbows, then place the back of your hands together, in front of your chest, flexing the wrist, and raising your elbows (Figure A.7). Hold these positions for 10 seconds and repeat 8 to 12 times.

After two to three weeks, wrist exercises can be started. You can do this by holding a light 3 to 5 pound dumbbell weight or grabbing a can of soup with your forearm on a counter top and your wrist dangling just over the edge of the counter. With your palm facing the floor and your elbow bent at 90 degrees, extend the wrist while holding the weight (or can) (Figure A.8) and repeat 10 to 15 times, increasing the number of

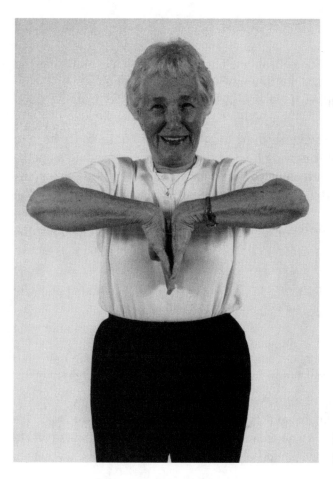

Figure A.7   Wrist flexion (reverse praying) stretch for tennis elbow.

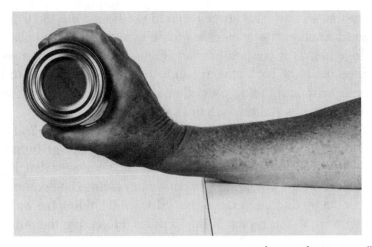

Figure A.8   Wrist extension exercise (using a can of soup) for tennis elbow.

repetitions as you become stronger. Then turn your hand so it faces the ceiling. Holding the weight, flex your wrist 10 to 15 times.

Surgery is considered a last resort and is done only if there is persistent pain and loss of function that lasts at least six months to a year. A common surgical procedure used for those with continued pain and disability consists of removing the scar tissue from the tendon, smoothing the bone, and reattaching the tendon. This is often done as an outpatient procedure. Recovery takes about 8 to 12 weeks.

Unfortunately Jerry did not stop playing tennis for more than a few days. The temptation to play just seemed to be too great. He kept reinjuring his elbow. Now 18 months later, he has chronic pain and has received three cortisone shots. He still tries to play an occasional doubles match, but avoids strong backhand returns.

Final Message

There is always a risk of injury when you exercise or participate in sports. However, the benefits of your training greatly outweigh those risks. Injury prevention, immediate treatment, and alternative exercises can reduce the time of inactivity and help you maintain your fitness.

Calculating your 1-repetition (1-RM) maximum weight

Max. # of Repetitions	Divide the Weight Lifted by
10	.73
9	.76
8	.79
7	.82
6	.85
5	.88
4	.91
3	.94
2	.97
1	1

Example: Karla can lift 100 pounds 8 times.
Her 1-RM is 100 lbs/.79 = 126.6 lb

My Strength-Training Workout Schedule

Photocopy these charts and use the exercise log to design your own workout.

Write in the lift and your 1-RM for that lift. Find these at the beginning of each four-week workout period. Example: (bench press) 110 pounds

(   ) _____lbs.   (   ) _____lbs
(   ) _____lbs.   (   ) _____lbs
(   ) _____lbs   (   ) _____lbs
(   ) _____lbs   (   ) _____lbs

Three days per week workout

Week # __	Day # __			Day # __			Day # __		
Exercise	**Weight**	**Sets**	**Repetitions**	**Weight**	**Sets**	**Repetitions**	**Weight**	**Sets**	**Repetitions**
Sample Bench Press	110 lb	3	8						

Week # __	Day # __ (light-moderate weight)			Day # __ (moderate weight)			Day # __ (light-moderate weight)		
Exercise	Weight	Sets	Repetitions	Weight	Sets	Repetitions	Weight	Sets	Repetitions

Week # __	Day # __ (light-moderate weight)			Day # __ (moderate weight)			Day # __ (light-moderate weight)		
Exercise	Weight	Sets	Repetitions	Weight	Sets	Repetitions	Weight	Sets	Repetitions

My Workout Schedule

Photocopy this chart and use the exercise log to record your aerobic exercise.

	1	2	3	4	5	6	7
Exercise type Exertion level Exercise time							
	8	9	10	11	12	13	14
Exercise type Exertion level Exercise time							
	15	16	17	18	19	20	21
Exercise type Exertion level Exercise time							
	22	23	24	25	26	27	28
Exercise type Exertion level Exercise time							
	29	30	31	Sample day Jogging 2/10 30 minutes			
Exercise type Exertion level Exercise time							

References

1. Exercise: The Best Medicine

Chishom DM, et al. Physical activity readiness. Br Columbia Med J 1975;17:375–378.

Goldberg L, Elliot E, editors. Exercise for Prevention and Treatment of Illness. F.A. Davis, Philadelphia, 1994.

U.S. Department of Health and Human Services. Physical activity and health. A report from the surgeon general. Atlanta: U.S. Department of Health and Human Services, Centers for Disease Control and Prevention, National Center for Chronic Disease Prevention and Health Promotion, 1996.

Passo M, et al. The ocular hypotensive effect of exercise conditioning in glaucoma suspects. Arch Ophthalmol 1991;109:1096–1098.

Butler RM, Goldberg L. Exercise and prevention of coronary heart disease. Primary Care Clinics of North America 1989;16:99–114.

Thune I, et al. Physical activity and the risk of breast cancer. N Engl J Med 1997;336:1269–1275.

2. Finding Your Way to Regular Exercise

Pate RR, et al. Physical activity and public health. JAMA 1995;273: 402–407. (Report of a panel of experts who reviewed the evidence for effects of regular physical activity. Based on that review, they drafted these recommendations. The advice has been endorsed by the Centers for Disease Control, the American College of Sports Medicine, the American Heart Association, and the National Institutes of Health.)

Prochaska JO, DeClemente CC. Stages and process of change in smoking: towards an integrative model of change. J Consult Clin Psychol 1983;51:390–395. (These investigators proposed the six stages of change, which have been confirmed to occur with many different behaviors. Their description, also called the 'transtheoretic model,' classifies an individual's stage and allows tailoring recommendations to be most productive.)

Marcus BH, Simkin LR. The transtheoretical model: applications to exercise behavior. Med Sci Sports Exerc 1994; 1400–1404. (Bess Marcus and colleagues have done the most work using the stages of change [the transtheoretic model] with exercise.)

Dishman RD, Buckworth J. Increasing physical activity: a quantitative synthesis. Med Sci Sports Exerc 1996;28:706–719. (This is a review article and more information can be found in Rod Dishman's book, Advances in Exercise Adherence, Champaign, Ill.: Human Kinetics; 1994. Unfortunately, despite all we know about what relates to adherence, it has not translated in ways to make it easy to get regular exercise.)

Miller WR, Rollnick S. Motivational Interviewing. New York: The Guilford Press; 1991. (This book includes chapters on ways to motivate change. The techniques were first used to help people stop drinking alcohol and using drugs. They also are effective when assisting people to make a good habit, as well as break a bad one.)

Sherman SE, Hershman WY. Exercise counseling: how do general internists do? J Gen Intern Med 1993;8:243–248. (Don't expect too much from your health care provider. Doctors usually do not counsel patients about exercise. Reasons that they do not were it never seems to work, no time to do it, do not know how to do it effectively, patients are not interested, and do not get reimbursed for it.)

3. Exercise for Bone Health

Gregg EW, et al. Physical activity and osteoporotic fracture risk in older women. Ann Intern Med 1998;129:81–88. (Researchers found that women who engage in moderate physical activity—which is achievable by most community dwelling elderly—reduced their risk of hip fracture.)

Nelson MR, et al. Effects of high-intensity strength training on multiple risk factors for osteoporotic fractures: a randomized controlled trial. JAMA 1994;272:1909–1914. (This was a year-long study of women who strength trained twice a week. When compared with matched women who did not exercise, the 20 who did had significantly increased strength, muscle mass, and dynamic balance. Their bone density increased by about 1 percent.)

Bailey DA, Faulkner RA, McKay HA. Growth, physical activity, and bone mineral acquisition. Exercise Sport Science Review 1996; 24:233–266.

National Osteoporosis Foundation at 1150 17th Street NW, Suite 500 Washington, D.C. 20038-4603. 202-223-0344 or 800-624-BONE; TTY 202-466-4315; E-mail: *orbdnrc@nof.org*. (This nonprofit organization was established in 1986. They have a catalog with educational materials. It can be obtained free at 202-223-2226.)

Bissinger M. Osteoporosis. An Exercise Guide. Workfit Consultants; 1998. (This brief guide divides exercises as resistance [bone strengthening], postural, and balance exercises. It also presents illustrated guides to lifting and body mechanics.)

Simkin A, Ayalon J. Bone Loading. London: Prion; 1997. (Paperback book with illustrations of exercises that load your bones to prevent osteoporosis.)

Exercise videos for those with osteoporosis are available through the web site *http://www.crm.mb.ca/scip/health/deerlo10.html*: Exercise Therapy for Osteoporosis and Postural Back Pain. Toronto: Canadian Learning Company, 1993; Osteoporosis Basic Exercise Program. Toronto: Osteoporosis Society of Canada, 1990; and Tai Chi for Elders. Toronto: Canadian Learning Company; 1990.

Menopause: A guide to smart choices. Consumer Reports 1999;64(1):50–54. (In a few years, we should have better information about the risks and benefits of estrogen replacement. This article presents what is currently known and how it relates to different types of hormone replacements.)

Office of Research on Women's Health was established to support the National Institutes of Health addressing the needs of women. *http://ohrm.od.nih.gov/orwh/women.html*

4. Exercise for Arthritis and Back Pain Relief

The National Institute of Arthritis and Musculoskeletal and Skin Diseases has informational pamphlets on different kinds of arthritis and their treatments, including exercise. A four-page listing of the Institute's offerings or specific pamphlets can be ordered by phone 301-496-8188; fax (301-587-4352); from its web site *http.//www.nig.gov/niams/*.

The Arthritis Foundation has information on all types of arthritis and their respective treatments. Their phone number is 1-800-283-7800, and their web site is *http.//www.arthritis.org/*. Look for Exercise and Your Arthritis (brochure # 835-5455).

Information on your aching feet and proper footwear can be obtained from the American Orthopedic Foot and Ankle Society at 1-800-235-4855. The American College of Foot and Ankle Surgeon also distributes pamphlets through their Foot Health Institute at 1-888-843-3338.

Sayce V, Fraser I. Exercise Beats Arthritis. Palo Alto, Cal.: Bull Publishing Company; 1998. (Majority of the book is specifics about different exercises, illustrated with over 200 pictures.) Also you can order Exercise Can Beat Arthritis and Exercise Can Beat Arthritis: Getting Stronger videotapes from View Video [1-800-VIEWVID; *http.//www.view.com*]).

Sammon, Patricia, YMCA of the USA. Healthy Back Book. Champaign, Ill.: Human Kinetics Publisher, Inc.; 1994. (Practical information about back anatomy, immediate care of back injuries, and useful exercises to prevent future back problems.)

Ettinger WH Jr, et al. A randomized trial comparing aerobic exercise and resistance exercise with a health education program in older adults with knee osteoarthritis. JAMA 1997;277:25–31. (Both types of exercise were beneficial for people with arthritis.)

Gordon NF. Arthritis: Your Complete Exercise Guide. Champaign, Ill.: Human Kinetics Publisher, Inc.; 1993.

McCain GA, et al. A controlled trial of the effects of a supervised cardiovascular fitness training program on the manifestations of primary fibromyalgia. Arthritis Rheum 1988;31:1135–1141. (Gradual aerobic conditioning benefitted people with fibromyalgia.)

Straight Talk on Spondylitis. The Spondylitis Association of America is a national nonprofit organization established in 1983 and a resource for all aspects of the disorder. Their number is 1-800-777-8189 or *http.//www.spondylitis.org*.

Deal CL, Moskowitz RW. Nutraceuticals as therapeutic agents in osteoarthritis. Rheumatic Disease Clinics of North America 1999;25: 379–395. (Review of studies concerning glucosamine and chontroitan use.)

Golden BD, Abramson SB. Selective Cyclooxytgenase-2 inhibitors. Rheumatic Disease Clinics of North America 1999;25:359–378. (Summary findings with the newer COX-2 selective NSAIDs.)

5. Exercise to Prevent and Treat Diabetes

Campaign, BN. Exercise in the management of diabetes mellitus. In: Goldberg L, Elliot D, editors. Exercise for Prevention and Treatment of Illness, Philadelphia: F.A. Davis; 1994. pp. 173–188.

Ericksson KF, Lindgarde F. Prevention of type 2 (non-insulin-dependent) diabetes mellitus by diet and physical exercise. *Diabetologia* 1991;34: 891–898.

Helmrich SP, et al. Physical activity and reduced occurrence of non-insulin-dependent diabetes mellitus. N Engl J Med 1991;325:147–152.

Kriska AM, Blair SN, Pereira MA. The potential role of physical activity in the prevention of non-insulin-dependent diabetes mellitus: the epidemiological evidence. In: Holloszy JO, editor. Exercise and Sport Sciences Reviews, Baltimore: Williams & Wilkins; 1994. pp. 121–143.

Ivy JL, Zderic TW, Foge DL. Prevention and treatment of non-insulin-dependent diabetes mellitus. In: Holloszy JL, editor. Exercise and Sport Sciences Reviews. Philadelphia: Lippincott, William, & Wilkins; 1999. pp. 1–35.

6. Exercise to Treat Abnormal Cholesterol Levels

Goldberg L, Elliot D. The use of exercise to improve lipid and lipoprotein levels. In: Goldberg L, Elliot D, editors. Exercise for Prevention and Treatment of Illness, Philadelphia: F.A. Davis; 1994. pp. 189–210.

Durstine JL, Haskell WL. Effects of exercise training on plasma lipids and lipoproteins. In: Holloszy J, editor. Exercise and Sport Sciences Reviews. Baltimore: Williams & Wilkins; Vol. 22, 1994. pp. 477–521.

Perrault S, et al. Treating hyperlipidemia for the primary prevention of coronary disease. Arch Intern Med 1998; 157:375–381.

Scandinavian Simvastatin Survival Study Group. Randomised trial of cholesterol lowering in 4,444 patients with coronary heart disease; the Scandinavian Simvistatin Survival Study (4S). Lancet 1994; 334:1383–1389.

Shepherd J, et al. Prevention of coronary heart disease with pravastatin in men with hypercholesterolemia. N Engl J Med 1995; 333:1301–1307.

Stefanick ML, et al. Effects of diet and exercise in men and post-menopausal women with low levels of HDL cholesterol. N Engl J Med 1998; 339:12–20.

7. Exercise to Lose Weight

Elliot DL, Goldberg L, Girard DE. Obesity: pathophysiology and practical management. J Gen Intern Med 1987;2:188–198.

Fatis M, et al. Following up on a commercial weight loss program: Do the pounds stay off after your picture has been in the newspaper? J Am Dietetic Assoc 1989;89:547–548. (Follow-up on 31 patients who lost weight and had their pictures in the paper revealed that 28 percent maintained the weight loss after 20 months. Almost half of those keeping the weight loss remained in the program, versus 5 percent of those who gained the weight back.)

Pi-Sunyer FX. Medical hazards of obesity. Ann Intern Med 1993;117:655–660. (Brief review of risks of obesity.)

Rosenbaum M, et al. Obesity. N Engl J Med 1997;337:396–406. (Review from August 1997).

The web has several sites that calculate your Body Mass Index. Point your browser toward the American Medical Associations's *http://www.ama-assn.org/insight/gen_hlth/pernutri/lessweig.htm* or the Chicago Tribune's *http://chitrib.webpoint.com/fitness/calburn.htm*.

Expert Panel on the Identification, Evaluation, and Treatment of Overweight and Obesity in Adults. Executive summary of the clinical guidelines on the identification, evaluation, and treatment of overweight and obesity in adults. Arch Intern Med 1998;158:1855–1867. (Exhaustive review by 115 experts about what works for weight loss; basically, it is change your eating and exercise. Also has the new criteria for obesity based on the Body Mass Index.)

Kingsbury BD. Full Figure Fitness. Life Enhancement Publications, ISBN 0-87322-923-1. (Sensible, easy-to-follow program, and the book also has lots of additional information on nutrition and weight loss.)

The National Institute on Diabetes and Digestive and Kidney Diseases at the National Institutes of Health offers publications and videos about medically sound weight loss and information on university-based weight-control programs at WIN (Weight Control Information); 1 Win Way; Bethesda, MD 20892-3665; phone 1-800-WIN-8098.

Studies by DASH (Dietary Approaches to Stop Hypertension) researchers have shown that a diet high in fruits and vegetables can reduce high-blood pressure quickly and safely without drugs. The DASH diet was not specifically designed to promote weight loss, but many participants shed pounds. This diet is a good starting point for overweight people who are unclear about what it means to eat a healthy diet. Information can be found at *http://dash.bwh. harvard.edu*

Shape Up America! is a national program dedicated to promoting safe, healthy weight loss through increased physical activity. Founded by former Surgeon General C. Everett Koop, M.D., its web site also helps you calculate your body mass index. It offers a library of weight-control materials, recipes, and evaluations of commercial and noncommercial weight-loss programs. It is at *http://www.shapeup.org/sua*

Dietary Guidelines for Americans is operated by the US Department of Agriculture. The site includes information about healthy nutrition and the diet recommended by government experts. It is at *http://www. nal.usda.gov/fnic/dga/dguide95.html*

There are several interactive web sites concerning weight loss. Examples include the following:

http://www.dietcity.com/

http://www.diettalk.com/

http://www.jennycraig.com/

http://www.learneducation.com/; phone 1-800-736-7323

http://www.niddk.nih.gov/health/nutrit/win.htm

http://www.weightwatchers.com/

8. Exercise to Lower Blood Pressure

Joint National Committee on Detection, Evaluation, and Treatment of High Blood Pressure. The sixth Report of the Joint National Committee on Prevention, Detection, Evaluation, and Treatment of High Blood Pressure. Arch Intern Med 1997;157:2413–2446.

Goldberg L, Elliot DL. Exercise as treatment for essential hypertension. In: Goldberg L, Elliot DL, editors. Exercise for Prevention and Treatment of Illness. Philadelphia: F.A. Davis;1994. pp. 27–47.

Tipton, CM. Exercise, training and hypertension: an update. In: Holloszy JO, editor. Exercise and Sport Sciences Reviews. Baltimore: Williams & Wilkins; 1991. Vol. 19, pp. 447–506.

Appel LJ, et al. (for the DASH Collaborative Research Group.) A clinical trial of the effects of dietary patterns on blood pressure. N Engl J Med. 1997;336:1117–1124.

Orbach P, Lowenthal DT. Evaluation and treatment of hypertension in active individuals. Med Sci Sports Exerc 1998;30 (10 Suppl)S354–S366.

Hayashi T, et al. Walking to work and risk of hypertension in men: the Osaka health survey. Ann Intern Med 1999;130:21–26.

9. Exercise to Prevent and Treat Heart Disease

Powell KE, et al. Physical activity and the incidence of coronary heart disease. Ann Rev Public Health 1987;8:253–287.

Lakka, TA, et al. Relation of leisure-time physical activity and cardiorespiratory fitness to the risk of acute myocardial infarction in men. N Engl J Med 1994;330:1549–1554.

Lee I, Hsieh C, Paffenbarger, R. Exercise intensity and longevity in men: the Harvard alumni health study. JAMA 1995;273:1179–1184.

Mittleman M, et al. Triggering of acute myocardial infarction by heavy physical exertion: Protection against triggering by regular exertion. N Engl J Med 1993;329:1677–1683.

Ekelund LG, et al. Physical fitness as a predictor of cardiovascular mortality in asymptomatic North American men: the Lipid Research Clinics Mortality Follow-up Study. N Engl J Med 1988; 319:1379–1384.

Peters RK, et al. Physical fitness and subsequent myocardial infarction in healthy workers. JAMA 1983;249:3052–3056.

Beniamini Y, et al. High-intensity strength training of patients enrolled in an outpatient cardiac rehabiliation program. J Cardiopulmonary Rehabil 1999:19(1):8–17.

Agnarsson U, et al. Effects of leisure-time physical activity and ventilatory function on risk for stroke in men. Ann Intern Med 1999; 130:987–992.

10. Exercise to Slow (and Reverse) Aging

Clark E. Growing Old Is Not for Sissies: Portraits of Senior Athletes. San Francisco, Cal.: Pomegranate Calendars and Books; 1990. (Pictures of elderly athletes; a second edition provides follow up on these inspiring athletes ten years after the original publication).

Clark J. Full Life Fitness. Champaign, Ill.: Human Kinetics Publishers; 1992. (Exercise programs for mature adults; Human Kinetics is probably the largest publisher of books concerning physical activity, and they carry programs tailored to all sorts of individuals (1-800-747-4457).

AAHPERD (American Alliance for Health, Physical Education, Recreation & Dance) has many publications, with several targeted for specific populations. Examples include: Mature Stuff: Activity for the Older Adults, and Who? Me? Exercise? Safe Exercise for People Over 50; for information call 1-800-213-7193.

AARP (American Association for Retired Persons) web site has links to many sites concerning aging and exercise. *http://www.sf.med.va.gov/medlib/aging.htm.*

ACSM position stands on exercise and physical activity for older adults. Medicine & Science in Sports & Exercise 1998;30:992–1008. (Reviews the data concerning aerobic activities, strength training, postural stability training and flexibility, making recommendations for each; separate sections review psychological benefits and exercise for frail individuals; it lists 248 references)

Fiatarone MA, et al. Exercise training and nutritional supplementation for physical frailty in very elderly people. N Engl J Med 1994; 330:1769–1775. (10-week study of 100 individuals; strength training [three times per week] improved strength and function; nutritional supplementation alone was no better than control.)

Campbell AJ, et al. Randomized controlled trial of a general practice programme of home based exercise to prevent falls in elderly women. Br Med J 1997;315:1065–1069. ('Tailored physical therapy'—leg strengthening and balance—that provided four home visits, with follow-up phone calls. It improved balance and reduced falls by almost 50 percent.)

Evans WJ. Exercise training guidelines for the elderly. Medicine & Science in Sports & Exercise 1999;31:12–17.

Kallinen M, Markku A. Aging, physical activity, and sports injuries. Sports Medicine 1995;20:41–52. (Tabulates studies comparing younger and older exercisers; this article primarily deals with injuries among elderly athletes; aging results in greater risk of musculoskeletal injuries.)

Rowe JW, Kahn RL. Successful Aging. New York: Pantheon Books; 1998.

Sit and Be Fit: 509-448-9438 (a Monday through Friday TV program for seniors, hosted by Mary Ann Wilson, R.N.; the program is fun and encouraging)

National Institute on Aging (NIA) has many free publications. Contact the NIA Information Center at 1-800-222-2225 or by email at *niainfo@access.digex.net*.

11. Exercise to Elevate Mood and Treat Anxiety and Depression

National Institute of Mental Health at 1-800-421-4211; write to National Institute of Mental Health, 5600 Fishers Lane, Room 7C02,

Rockville, MD, 20857; call 301-443-4513 for program/materials; or visit the NIMH's web site at *http://www.nimh.nih.gov*.

Sheehan, DV, M.D. The Anxiety Disease. New York: Bantam Books; 1986; (Sheehan covers the seven progressive stages of the disease, and the causes, treatment, and recovery, using case histories as examples. The book also contains an anxiety scale to help you determine whether the level of your anxiety is excessive; list price: $6.50, ISBN: 0553272454.)

Cronkite, K. On the Edge of Darkness: Conversations about Conquering Depression. New York: Dell Publishing; 1995. (Kathy Cronkite is Walter Cronkite's daughter. She interviews well-known people about their depression, discusses her own depression, and presents information about the disorder; list price: $13.95, ISBN: 0385314264.)

Papolos, D, Papolos J. Overcoming Depression: The Definitive Resource for Patients and Families Who Live with Depression and Manic-Depression. New York: HarperCollins; 1997. (list price: $15.00, ISBN: 0060927828.)

12. Your Personal Exercise Prescription

Roitman JL, editor. ACSM's Resource Manual for Guidelines for Exercise Testing and Prescription, 3rd ed. Baltimore: Williams & Wilkins; 1998.

Goldberg L, Elliot EL, Exercise. In: Dornbrand L, Hoole AJ, Fletcher RH, editors. Manual of Clinical Problems in Adult Ambulatory Care. 3rd ed. Lippincott-Raven (publisher); Philadephia: Lippincott-Raven; 1997. pp. 689–694.

Afterword

Goldberg L, et al. Managing exercise-related injuries in older adults. Patient Care 1999;33(11):74–87.

Sparling PB, Millard-Stafford M. Keeping sports participants safe in hot weather. The Physican and Sports Medicine 1999;27(7):27–34.

Colville MR. Rehabilitation of orthopedic injuries. In: Exercise for Prevention and Treatment of Illness. pp. 128–152. Goldberg L, Elliot D. (editors). Philadelphia, PA.: F.A. Davis; 1994.

Index

Page numbers followed by an f indicate a figure; page numbers followed by a t indicate a table.

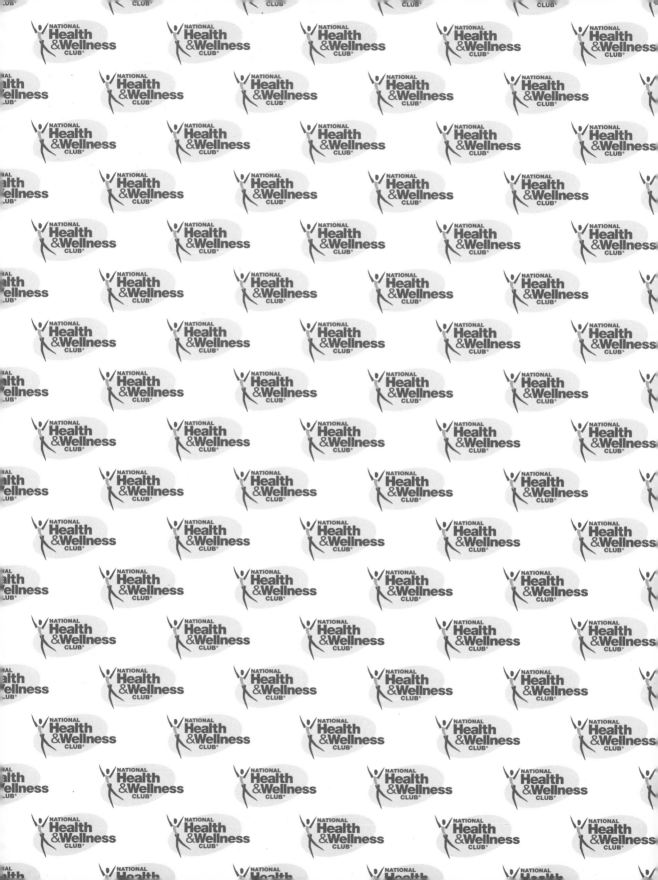